Nursing Care

In

Internal Medicine

The Complete Guide

ALEXANDRE CAREWELL

Table of contents

« In internal medicine, each patient is a universe in itself, and our mission is to navigate their inner galaxies to restore balance and health. »

Introduction:

The importance of internal medicine.

Internal medicine, often considered to be the art of deduction and the very essence of medicine, occupies a central position in the overall care of the patient. Its specificity lies in its ability to encompass all pathologies, whether common or rare, and to understand the patient as a whole, both physically and psychologically.

First, let's look at its origins. Historically, internal medicine was born out of a desire to understand and treat diseases in their entirety, without limiting itself to one organ or one speciality. It is a discipline that thrives on complexity, that thrives on enigmatic cases and that delights in deciphering the mysteries of the human body. It is a reflection of the inexhaustible curiosity of doctors, of their determination always to seek, to understand and, above all, to treat.

Internal medicine is the hub around which many other specialities revolve. It favours a holistic approach, in which every symptom, every sign, is a piece of a complex puzzle. The internist is often seen as a medical detective, gathering clues, hypothesising and drawing on a wealth of knowledge to make a precise diagnosis. The aim is not simply to treat a disease, but to understand the patient as a whole, to perceive the intricacies between the body's different systems and to detect subtle imbalances.

But beyond this quest for diagnosis, internal medicine also embodies a profoundly humanist philosophy. It reminds us of the importance of the doctor-patient relationship, based on trust, listening and respect. In an increasingly technological and specialised medical world, the internist remains the guardian of the indefectible link between science and humanity.

The importance of internal medicine can also be seen in its ability to evolve and adapt to the new challenges of our time. Faced with emerging diseases and pathologies that are becoming increasingly complex as a result of medical advances and rising life expectancy, internists are on the front line, ready to decipher, learn and innovate.

Internal medicine is not just another medical speciality; it is a state of mind, a vocation and, for many, a passion. It reminds us that behind every illness there is an individual, with his or her fears, hopes and uniqueness. And it is in this profound recognition of the individual that the true art of medicine lies.

The changing role of the nurse in this department.

The role of the nurse in internal medicine, as in other areas of healthcare, has undergone major changes over the years. These developments have been driven not only by technological and medical advances, but also by social, ethical and legislative changes.

In the past, nurses were seen mainly as people who carried out tasks, as assistants to the doctor. Their role was limited to specific tasks: administering basic care, ensuring the patient's cleanliness and comfort, and scrupulously following medical prescriptions. It was a time when the medical hierarchy was rigid, and nurses had little room for manoeuvre.

Over time, the nursing profession has gained in recognition and autonomy. This development has been driven by a number of factors. Firstly, nurse training has become denser, incorporating more in-depth knowledge of anatomy, physiology and pharmacology, as well as the human sciences. This has given nurses the tools they need to adopt a more clinical and analytical approach to their practice.

In the field of internal medicine, the complexity of cases, the heterogeneity of pathologies and the need for comprehensive care have led nurses to broaden their field of action. Nurses have become pivotal members of the medical team, working closely with doctors, pharmacists, social workers and other healthcare professionals.

The modern internal medicine nurse has a strong assessment capacity, capable of rapidly identifying changes in the patient's clinical condition, taking the initiative and adapting care accordingly. Their role is no longer limited to simply carrying out tasks, but encompasses planning, patient education, prevention and even research.
The nurse-patient relationship has also evolved. Nurses are now more involved in the decision-making process, accompanying patients and their families, educating them about the disease and treatments, and helping them to make informed decisions.

Finally, technological advances, the rise of telemedicine and the emphasis on home care have also influenced the role of the internal medicine nurse. These changes have opened up new horizons and created new opportunities, but also challenges in terms of adaptability and continuing education.

Today's internal medicine nurse is a clinician, an educator, a researcher and a defender of patients' rights. A remarkable development, reflecting the dynamism and richness of this profession, which is essential to our healthcare system.

Chapter 1:
UNDERSTANDING INTERNAL MEDICINE

What is internal medicine?

Internal medicine is a medical speciality dedicated to the prevention, diagnosis, management and treatment of adult diseases. It is distinguished by its comprehensive, holistic approach to the patient, focusing not on a particular organ or type of pathology, but on the individual as a whole.

Here are some key points about internal medicine:

Holistic approach: Internists, who specialise in internal medicine, are interested in the whole human body. They are trained to treat patients with a number of concomitant conditions and try to understand how these conditions may interact with each other.

Range of diseases: Internists treat a wide range of diseases, from the most common to the rarest. This includes, but is not limited to, cardiac, respiratory, digestive, renal, endocrine and haematological diseases.

Prevention and education: Internal medicine is not just about treating illness; it also focuses on prevention. Internists play a crucial role in screening for disease, providing vaccinations, promoting a healthy lifestyle and educating patients about their state of health.

Role of coordinator: In complex pathologies requiring the intervention of several specialists, the internist can act as a coordinator, ensuring that the patient receives coherent and comprehensive care.

Rigorous training: To become an internist, a doctor must undergo rigorous postgraduate training, often followed by sub-specialisation in fields such as cardiology, gastroenterology, rheumatology, etc.

Complex diagnosis: Thanks to their training and global approach, internists are often called upon to help diagnose complex or enigmatic cases.

Continuing Care: Internists can provide care throughout an adult's life, from adolescence to old age, enabling a deep and lasting understanding of the patient's medical history.

Internal medicine is a vast and varied speciality, centred on the individual, encompassing the whole range of adult ailments and emphasising a global, integrative approach. Internists are often described as "doctors' doctors" because of their expertise in diagnosing and treating complex diseases.

History and development.

The history of internal medicine is rich and fascinating, reflecting advances in medicine itself, social developments and the challenges faced by the medical profession over the centuries. Let's take a look at the history of this speciality.

Origins:

Antiquity: From ancient times, doctors such as Hippocrates in Greece adopted a holistic approach to the patient, seeking to understand illness in the context of the individual and his or her environment. This was the genesis of what we might think of as internal medicine.

Middle Ages: During this period, medicine was mainly taught in religious institutions. Medical knowledge was based on ancient texts, and the clinical approach was largely dominated by humoral theories.

The emergence of Modern Internal Medicine:

Renaissance: This period saw a renewed interest in science and human anatomy. The art of auscultation and palpation was developed, laying the foundations for clinical examination.

19th century: The development of scientific methods and the advent of microbiology revolutionised our understanding of disease. Internal medicine, as we know it, began to take shape. Hospitals became centres of education and research.

20th century: With the discovery of antibiotics, internal medicine saw its treatment capabilities expand considerably. Technological advances, such as medical imaging, enhanced diagnosis. The speciality was subdivided into numerous sub-specialities (cardiology, nephrology, endocrinology, etc.), reflecting the growing complexity of medicine.

Contemporary challenges:

21st century: The beginning of this century was marked by the explosion of knowledge in genetics and molecular biology, offering targeted therapeutic prospects. Internal medicine must also respond to new challenges such as an ageing population, chronic diseases, antibiotic resistance and the growing importance of prevention.

Personalised medicine: With advances in genomics, internal medicine is at the forefront of efforts to offer personalised care, tailored to the genetic and biological particularities of each individual.

The history of internal medicine is that of a never-ending quest to understand and treat disease in its broadest context. It bears witness to the evolution of our conception of health and disease, and continues to reinvent itself in the face of contemporary challenges. It is a speciality which, while embracing technological and scientific advances, remains firmly rooted in the art of medicine: listening to, understanding and caring for the individual in all his or her complexity.

The main diseases and conditions treated.

Internal medicine covers a broad spectrum of diseases and conditions. Given its global and holistic approach, the internist is often faced with complex cases involving several organ systems. Here is an overview of the main diseases and conditions frequently treated by internists:

Cardiovascular:
- Hypertension
- Heart failure
- Coronary heart disease
- Arrhythmias
- Peripheral vascular diseases

Lung:
- Asthma
- Chronic bronchitis and emphysema
- Pneumonia
- Tuberculosis
- Idiopathic pulmonary fibrosis

Gastrointestinal:
- Peptic ulcer disease
- Inflammatory bowel diseases (Crohn's disease, ulcerative colitis)
- Hepatitis
- Cirrhosis
- Diseases of the pancreas

Renal:

      Chronic renal   failure

      Glomerulonephritis

      Diabetic nephropathy

      Renal   lithiasis

Endocrine:

      Type 1 and type 2 diabetes

      Hyperthyroidism and hypothyroidism

      Diseases of the adrenal   glands

      Osteoporosis

Haematological:

      Anemias of various origins (iron deficiency, megaloblastic, haemolytic)

      Thrombosis and embolisms

      Leukaemia and lymphoma

Infectious diseases:

      Respiratory infections (pneumonia, bronchitis)

      Urinary tract infections

      Endocarditis

      Sepsis and septic shock

      HIV/AIDS

Rheumatology:

      Rheumatoid   arthritis

      Systemic   lupus erythematosus

      Ankylosing spondylitis

      Drops and pseudodrops

Autoimmune and systemic diseases:

      Sjögren 's syndrome

      Scleroderma

      Vasculitis

Electrolytics and metabolic disorders:

      Sodium, potassium and calcium imbalances

      Acidosis and alkalosis

It is important to note that internal medicine is not limited to these diseases. Internists are trained to treat a wide range of conditions and are often called upon to make complex or enigmatic diagnoses. What's more, as medicine evolves, new pathologies or new variants of existing diseases regularly emerge, requiring constant updating of knowledge.

The players in internal medicine :
The role of the internist

The internist, or simply internist, plays a crucial role in modern medicine. Renowned for their ability to treat complex diseases and make diagnoses in enigmatic cases, internists are distinguished by their holistic approach to patient care. Here is a detailed overview of their main tasks:

Diagnostic expert:
> Internists are often seen as "medical detectives". They are called upon to diagnose complex, atypical or rare conditions.
> It uses a combination of interviews, clinical examinations and paraclinical investigations to establish a precise diagnosis.

Chronic Disease Management:
> Internists often manage patients with chronic diseases such as diabetes, hypertension and cardiovascular disease, among others.
> It is responsible for adjusting treatments, educating patients and preventing complications.

Care Coordination:
> In cases where several specialists are involved in the treatment, the internist often acts as coordinator, ensuring continuity and consistency of care.

Holistic approach:
> The internist looks beyond symptoms and illnesses to the patient as a whole, including

history, lifestyle, concerns and psychosocial needs.

Prevention and education:

Internists play an active role in disease prevention, particularly through vaccinations, screening and lifestyle advice.

He also educates patients about their condition, helping them to understand their illness and treatment.

Research and Evolution:

Many internists are involved in clinical research, seeking to improve diagnostic methods, therapeutic strategies and understanding of diseases.

They are also involved in training future doctors, sharing their expertise and experience.

Hospital consultation:

In a hospital setting, internists may be asked to give their opinion on patients admitted by other specialities, particularly when the diagnosis is uncertain or the management is complex.

The internist is a central pillar of modern medicine, combining vast medical knowledge with a patient-centred approach. Their ability to see the "big picture" while focusing on the details makes them a key player, whether in clinics, hospitals or universities.

The crucial importance of the nurse.

Nurses occupy a fundamental position in healthcare. As the linchpin of the system, they not only implement medical treatments, but also play a central role in the physical, emotional and social well-being of patients. Let's take a look at the crucial importance of nurses in the medical landscape.

Direct Patient Care :
Nurses provide direct care, whether it's administering medication, monitoring vital signs, carrying out wound care or meeting patients' basic needs.

Patient Advocacy:
They act as patient advocates, ensuring that patients' rights are respected, that their concerns are heard, and that they receive the best possible care.

Liaison between Patients and the Medical Team :
The nurses act as a bridge between the patient and the rest of the medical team, ensuring smooth communication and coordinated care.

Education and Prevention :
They educate patients and their families about their state of health, medication, post-hospital care, disease prevention and health promotion.

Emotional   Support :
The human aspect of nursing care is invaluable. Nurses offer emotional support to patients and their families, particularly at critical or vulnerable times.

Leadership role :
Many nurses hold leadership positions, supervising other medical   staff, managing units or departments, or contributing to decision-making at institutional level.

Clinical Research :
Nurses are also involved in research, seeking to improve care practices, develop new methodologies or evaluate the effectiveness of interventions.

Global Vision of Care :
>   Unlike other healthcare professionals who may focus on a specific aspect of treatment, nurses have a holistic view of the patient, enabling them to anticipate needs, detect potential complications and ensure continuity of care.

Adaptability :
>   The world of healthcare is constantly changing, and nurses are often at the cutting edge, adapting to new technologies, methodologies and emerging challenges.

Ethics and Professional Integrity :
>   The nursing profession is guided by a strict code of ethics, ensuring that care is provided with compassion, respect for dignity and integrity.

The importance of nurses cannot be underestimated. They are the beating heart of many care homes, offering a unique blend of clinical skills, empathy and dedication. Their role extends far beyond the medical setting, touching, influencing and improving the lives of millions of people every day.

Chapter 2:
A TYPICAL DAY IN THE LIFE OF A NURSE IN INTERNAL MEDICINE

Start the day:

Starting the day is often seen as a defining moment that can influence the course of the following hours. A good start to the day can bring energy, concentration and positivity, while a chaotic morning can have the opposite effect. Here's a look at the importance of getting the day off to a good start, and some tips for creating beneficial morning rituals.

Dawn throws the first rays of light through the curtains, gently caressing the face of the sleeping man. The world outside gradually awakens, with the songs of birds, the hum of cars in the distance, and the murmur of the first footsteps of neighbours. It's these first moments, when the world shifts from darkness to light, that have the potential to set the tone for the whole day.

The Importance of the First Hour :

Tone for the Day: How we start our morning can often define our mood, energy level and mindset for the rest of the day.

Moment of Calm: Before the day becomes too chaotic, the morning often offers a moment of tranquillity where you can refocus, meditate or simply enjoy the solitude.

Opportunity   to Set Intentions: The early hours are the perfect time to set goals and intentions for the day, which can act as a compass to guide our actions and decisions.

Tips for a good start to the day:

Avoid Technology: Rather than immediately jumping on your phone or computer, take a few minutes to stretch, breathe deeply or simply be present.

Morning ritual: Establish a morning routine, whether it's meditation, writing, exercise or even a skincare ritual. These habits can help you start the day on the right foot.

Healthy eating: A nutritious, balanced breakfast can provide the energy you need to start the day with vitality.

Planning: Spend a few minutes reviewing your tasks for the day. This will help clarify your priorities and give you a sense of organisation going into the day.

Positivity: Cultivate a positive attitude first thing in the morning. Whether it's gratitude, reading an inspirational quote or listening to a happy song, find what makes you tick.

Starting the day is not simply a transition from sleep to wakefulness. It's an opportunity, a blank canvas on which to paint our hopes, dreams and intentions. With a little awareness and effort, every morning can become a harmonious prelude to a memorable day.

Transmission : ensure continuity of care.

Communication, often called "handover" in the medical context, is crucial to ensuring continuity and quality of care. They are moments when information, knowledge and experience are shared between healthcare professionals to ensure optimal patient care. Let's take a look at why communication is so essential and how it directly influences the quality of care.

The Nature of Transmissions :
Information is at the heart of communication. This can range from a simple mention of a patient's temperature to a complete summary of their clinical condition, history, care provided and recommendations for the coming hours or days.

Why are they Crucial? :

Continuity of care: Transmission ensures that the next professional to take over has all the information needed to continue care without interruption or omission.

Patient safety: omitting crucial information can lead to medical errors. Accurate and complete transmission helps to reduce the risks.

Efficient time management: By having a clear view of the patient's condition from the start of their shift, healthcare professionals can prioritise their interventions and manage their time effectively.

Team-building: Transmission promotes team cohesion. They are a time for exchange and collaboration, reinforcing the sense of belonging and team dynamics.

Principles of Effective Transmission :

Clarity: Information must be presented concisely and clearly to avoid any ambiguity.

Completeness: All relevant aspects of the patient's management must be covered, from the drugs administered to behavioural observations.

Structure: A structured transmission, often following a format or checklist, ensures that no important elements are omitted.

Interactivity: It's not just about talking, but also about listening. The professionals receiving the transmission must be given the opportunity to ask questions or seek clarification.

Documentation: In addition to oral transmission, having written documentation, such as notes or reports, can serve as a reference and ensure traceability.

Confidentiality: The information shared during communications is often sensitive. It is crucial to ensure that these exchanges remain confidential.

Communication is much more than a simple routine or formal procedure. They are the glue that binds the actions of multiple professionals around a patient's well-being. Ensuring their quality and effectiveness is essential to guaranteeing the safety and continuity of care. In an increasingly complex medical world, the ability to communicate effectively and accurately has become an invaluable skill.

Reviewing medical records: preparation and anticipation.

Reviewing medical records is an essential step in a patient's care. It provides a complete picture of a patient's medical history, current treatments and future needs. This process requires rigour, preparation and anticipation. Let's delve into the world of this task, which is so crucial to medical care.

Why is it important to prepare the medical records review properly?

Medical History: Understanding a patient's medical history is crucial to future decision-making. Everything from allergies and past surgeries to current treatments can influence the care plan.

Ensuring patient safety: An inappropriate or incomplete review can lead to medical errors. Careful preparation reduces the risks associated with missing or misinterpreted information.

Optimising time: With the time constraints often faced by healthcare professionals, a well-prepared review allows decisions to be taken quickly and efficiently.

Preparing for the Review :

Gathering information: Make sure you have all the relevant documents: hospital records, test results, notes from previous consultations, etc.

Chronological filing: Organise documents chronologically, from the oldest to the most recent, to make it easier to understand the patient's progress.

Highlighting Key Information: Underline or note the key points to remember for each document.

Prepare your Tools: Have tools such as pens, post-it notes or highlighters to hand for annotating and marking points of interest.

Anticipating needs and questions :

List of questions: Before the review, prepare a list of questions or points of clarification based on the information you have gathered.

Consult the Medical   Protocols: For specific conditions or treatments, familiarise yourself with the latest protocols or medical recommendations to anticipate the patient's needs.

Interdisciplinary collaboration: Anticipate the specialists or other health professionals who may be needed to provide comprehensive care.

After the Review :

Summary: Write a brief summary of key information to facilitate future management and communication with other professionals.

File Update: If new information has been discovered or changes have been made to the care plan, be sure to update the patient's medical file accordingly.

Communication: Share relevant information with the medical team and other professionals involved.

The review of medical records is a delicate dance between the medical past, the clinical present and the anticipation of the future. This task, although often perceived as administrative, is at the heart of medical care. By approaching this responsibility with rigour, preparation and anticipation, healthcare professionals can ensure they offer their patients optimal care.

Administering treatments:
Oral and intravenous drugs,
and subcutaneous.

Medicines are an essential part of medical treatment. They can be administered by various routes, depending on their formulation, therapeutic objective and the patient's clinical situation. Among these routes of administration, oral, intravenous and subcutaneous are among the most common. Let's take a look at the particularities of each of these routes and their implications for carers.

1. Oral medications :

Description: These are medicines administered by mouth, which then pass into the digestive system. They may take the form of tablets, capsules, syrups or suspensions.

Advantages: easy to administer, suitable for long-term treatment, generally low cost.

Disadvantages: Passage through the liver (first-pass effect), possible interactions with food, need for good patient compliance.

Precautions: Make sure the patient is able to swallow, be aware of contraindications and drug interactions.

2. Intravenous (IV) drugs :

Description: direct administration into a vein, usually via a catheter. This may be a bolus (rapid injection) or an infusion (over a longer period).

Advantages: rapid onset of action, precise dosage, possibility of administering large volumes or irritating drugs.

Disadvantages: Risk of infection, requires a sterile technique, potential complications associated with the venous route (thrombosis, phlebitis).

Precautions: Appropriate training for the insertion and management of venous lines, regular monitoring of the insertion site, compliance with asepsis protocols.

3. Subcutaneous drugs :

Description: Injection into the subcutaneous tissue, just below the skin. Commonly used for insulin or anticoagulants, for example.

Advantages: Relatively simple administration, predictable absorption, suitable for home use with self-injection.

Disadvantages: Limited volume of administration, possible local reactions (redness, pain).

Precautions: Rotation of injection sites to avoid lipoatrophy or lipohypertrophy, appropriate administration technique to minimise the risk of local reactions.

Implications for carers:

Training and competence: Carers must be trained and competent in the administration of drugs by different routes, understanding the advantages, disadvantages and precautions involved.

Patient education: In some cases, particularly for subcutaneous self-injection, carers have the role of educating and training the patient or their carers in the administration technique.

Monitoring: After administration, monitoring is often necessary to detect and manage any side effects or complications.

Each route of administration has its own specificities. Caregivers, whether nurses, pharmacists or doctors, must master these aspects to ensure effective and safe therapy. Understanding the pharmacokinetic and pharmacodynamic characteristics, as well as ongoing training, are essential to optimising the therapeutic benefits and minimising the risks for patients.

The challenges of multiple diseases.

Treating a patient suffering from several pathologies - or co-morbidities - is one of the major challenges facing healthcare professionals, particularly in internal medicine departments. Multiple conditions can lead to complications in care management, increase the risk of hospitalisation, and negatively influence the patient's quality of life. Let's take a look at the associated challenges and strategies for dealing with them.

1. Drug interactions :

Patients suffering from multiple diseases are often undergoing several treatments at the same time. This increases the risk of drug interactions, which can reduce the effectiveness of the drugs or cause adverse reactions.

2. Polypharmacy :

Polypharmacy, or taking a large number of medicines, can make it difficult for patients to comply with their treatment and increase the risk of medication errors.

3. Synergy of symptoms :
   The symptoms of different illnesses can reinforce each other. For example, depression can intensify the perception of pain in a patient suffering from arthritis.
4. Diagnostic complexity :
   The symptoms of different diseases can overlap, making diagnosis more complex.
5. Care coordination :
   A patient suffering from multiple pathologies may need to consult a number of different specialists. Ensuring effective coordination and transparent communication between these professionals is essential, but sometimes complex.
6. Impact on Quality of Life :
   Multiple pathologies can limit physical activity, affect mental health and reduce independence, profoundly affecting the patient's quality of life.

Strategies to overcome these challenges :
   Patient Centred   Approach :
      Understanding the patient's   n e e d s , concerns and priorities is essential to developing an individualised care plan.
   Regular Drug Review:
      It is crucial to regularly   r e v i e w   t h e patient's medication list to reduce polypharmacy and minimise the risk of drug interactions.
   Interprofessional Communication :
      Promoting open communication between all the professionals involved in a patient's care leads to better coordination and more comprehensive care.
   Education and Support :
      Informing patients and their families about their illnesses, treatments and symptom management helps to improve patient compliance and quality of life.

Using Technology :
> Digital tools, such as electronic medical records, can make it easier to coordinate care and monitor patients.

Close follow-up :
> Regular visits enable ongoing assessment of the patient's condition, adjustment of treatments and early detection of complications.

Caring for patients with multiple conditions requires a holistic, patient-centred approach that takes into account the complexity of their situation. With particular attention to coordination, communication and education, it is possible to offer quality care to these patients, thereby improving their health and well-being.

Patient follow-up : Clinical observations.

Clinical observation is a fundamental pillar of medical practice. It is the first step in the diagnostic and therapeutic approach and provides valuable insight into the patient's condition. In an internal medicine department, where patients may present with a variety of complex symptoms and co-morbidities, clinical observation is particularly essential. Let's take a closer look at this concept.

1. What is clinical observation?
Clinical observation is a systematic process by which the carer gathers information about the patient through direct observation. This may include physical examination, but also observation of behaviour, interactions, gait and other elements.

2. The components of clinical observation :

General examination: Assessment of the patient's general condition, level of consciousness, skin colour, morphology, etc.

Physical examination: Systematic examination of various parts of the body (auscultation, palpation, percussion).

Behavioural observation: Study of facial expressions, gait, movements and overall behaviour.

Observation of vital signs: Measurement of blood pressure, heart rate, respiratory rate, temperature, etc.

3. The importance of clinical observation in internal medicine :

Making an initial diagnosis: Many clinical signs can point to a specific disease or underlying condition.

Monitoring the progress of a disease: Repeated observations can be used to assess the progression of a disease or the effectiveness of a treatment.

Detecting abnormalities: Some subtle clinical signs may be early indicators of complications or new pathologies.

4. Challenges associated with clinical observation :

Subjective interpretation: Two clinicians may interpret an observation differently, especially if it is subtle.

Variability of symptoms: In internal medicine, the multiplicity of diseases and their varied presentation can make clinical observation more complex.

5. Optimising clinical observation :

Ongoing training: Carers must regularly update their knowledge and skills in clinical examination.

Use of standardised tools: Certain tools or scales can help to objectify certain observations.

Teamwork: Regularly discussing observations with other team members can help to gain a more complete and objective view.

Clinical observation is an essential skill in internal medicine, requiring special attention, ongoing training and a collaborative approach. Not only does it enable a diagnosis to be made, it also enables the progress of the disease to be monitored, treatments to be adjusted and complications to be prevented.

Communication
with the patient and their family.

Communication with patients and their families is one of the most crucial skills for an internal medicine healthcare professional. It influences not only the patient's understanding of their illness and treatment, but also their satisfaction, adherence to therapy and, ultimately, their health outcomes. In internal medicine departments, where diagnoses can be complex and treatments multifactorial, this communication is all the more essential.

1. The importance of effective communication :
  Trust and the therapeutic relationship: Good communication builds trust between patient, family and carer, which is essential for a successful therapeutic relationship.
  Informed decision-making: Patients need to understand their disease, their treatment options and the associated benefits and risks in order to make informed decisions.
  Reducing anxiety: Illness can be a source of anxiety. Clear, empathetic communication can help reduce this anxiety.
2. Effective Communication Techniques :
  Active listening: This involves paying full attention to what the patient or their family is saying, reflecting, clarifying and reformulating where necessary.

Simple, clear language: Avoid medical jargon and ensure that information is presented in an understandable way.

Non-verbal communication: take into account body language, eye contact and tone of voice.

Open questioning: Encourage patients to express themselves by asking open questions.

Validation of understanding: Regularly checking that the patient or their family has understood the information provided.

3. Tackling Sensitive Subjects :

There may be times when difficult news needs to be communicated, such as a serious diagnosis or an unfavourable disease progression.

Preparation: Anticipate emotional reactions and plan a quiet, private place for the discussion.

Empathy: Recognising and validating the emotions of patients and their families.

Honesty: It is essential to be both transparent and sensitive.

4. Involving the Family :

The family often plays a key role in the care and support of the patient.

Recognition: Recognising the role of the family and validating it as a partner in care.

Confidentiality: Ensuring confidentiality while sharing relevant information with the family.

Support: Providing resources or guidance if the family needs help managing the stress or anxiety associated with the illness.

5. Managing difficult situations :

There may be times when the patient or family is angry, frustrated or at odds with the medical team.

Stay calm: Don't react emotionally, but actively listen to their concerns.

Clarify: Often, dissatisfaction stems from a misunderstanding. Clarifying information can solve many problems.

Seeking a compromise: If possible, work together to find a solution acceptable to all parties.

Effective communication is at the heart of internal medicine, and it is essential for healthcare professionals to constantly develop and refine their communication skills. Successful communication can improve not only patient care, but also patient and family satisfaction, leading to better overall outcomes.

Chapter 3:
ESSENTIAL CLINICAL SKILLS

Clinical assessment :
The importance of the history.

The history, which refers to all the information gathered by the healthcare professional when questioning the patient, plays a central role in medical practice, particularly in internal medicine. It represents the first stage in the diagnostic process, guiding subsequent steps such as the physical examination, investigations and therapeutic decisions.

1. The history as a basis for diagnosis :
   Symptoms: The main symptoms that led the patient to seek help, how they started, how they developed, their characteristics, their intensity, and what aggravates or relieves them.
   Medical history: Previous illnesses, surgical procedures, allergies, current or recent treatments.
   Family history: The medical history of family members can provide clues to hereditary diseases or genetic predispositions.
2. More than just a list of symptoms:
   Context of onset: Understanding the context in which symptoms appear can help determine their cause.
   Influence on daily life: The effects of symptoms on the patient's ability to carry out daily activities.
   Feelings and emotions: Anxiety, stress, depression and other emotional states can influence, or be influenced by, medical conditions.

. The Art of Asking the Right Questions :

Opening technique: Start with open-ended questions, such as "What can I do for you today?" or "Tell me about your symptoms."

Avoid suggesting answers: Ask questions in a neutral way to elicit a genuine response from the patient.

Targeted questioning: If necessary, ask more specific questions to clarify certain points.

4. The Importance of Active Listening: Listening is just as important as questioning. Active listening involves concentrating fully, understanding, responding and remembering what the patient is saying.

5. The challenges of history-taking :

Reluctant or distrustful patients: Some patients may be reluctant to share intimate details or may fear being judged.

Language or cultural barriers: It is essential to understand and respect the patient's cultural beliefs and, if necessary, to use an interpreter.

Complexity of symptoms: In internal medicine, patients may present with a range of seemingly unrelated symptoms. The history must be thorough enough to capture this complexity.

6. Impact on Patient Care :

Diagnostic insight: A complete and accurate history is often the key to making a correct diagnosis.

Treatment planning : Understanding the patient's needs, concerns and life context can guide treatment decisions.

The history is not a mere formality, but a powerful diagnostic tool. It requires the clinician to combine technical skill with intuition, empathy and listening. In internal medicine, with the diversity and complexity of cases, it is all the more essential. It lays the foundations for patient-centred, appropriate and effective management.

Carrying out a clinical examination.

The clinical examination is a fundamental stage in the medical assessment, following the medical history. It involves a systematic assessment of the patient using the clinician's senses, sometimes aided by a few simple tools, such as the stethoscope or reflex hammer. The aim of this examination is to confirm or refute the diagnostic hypotheses put forward on the basis of the history.

1. Preparing for the Clinical Examination :
   Create the right environment: Make sure the room is well lit, warm and private.

   Explanation and consent: Always inform the patient of what you are going to do and why, and obtain their consent.

   Positioning the patient: Make sure that the patient is comfortably seated, depending on the part of the body to be examined.

2. General review :
   General appearance: Note state of consciousness, complexion, posture, level of anxiety or pain.

   Vital signs: Temperature, pulse, blood pressure, respiratory rate, oxygen saturation.

   Skin examination: colour, texture, elasticity, presence of rashes, bruises, scars or lumps.

3. Systematic examination by device :
   Cardiovascular examination: Auscultation of the heart, palpation of peripheral pulses, checking for oedema of the lower limbs.

   Respiratory examination: Inspection, palpation, percussion and auscultation of the lungs.

   Abdominal examination: Inspection, auscultation, percussion and palpation of the abdomen.

- **Neurological examination**: Assessment of consciousness, cranial nerves, muscle strength, reflexes, coordination and sensation.
- **Musculoskeletal examination**: Assessment of mobility, strength and stability of joints, looking for pain or deformity.
- **ENT and ophthalmology examination**: Examination of the throat, ears, nose and eyes.
- **Examination of the genital, urinary and rectal systems:** According to symptoms and with the patient's consent.

4. Examination techniques :
- **Inspection**: Visual observation of different parts of the body.
- **Palpation**: Using the hands to feel the texture, size, shape, consistency and location of certain parts of the body.
- **Percussion**: Lightly tap the surface of the body to determine the density of the underlying organs.
- **Auscultation**: Listening to the sounds produced by the heart, lungs, abdomen and other organs.

5. Importance of Observation and Clinical Intuition :
- **Subtle signs**: Sometimes, discreet clinical signs can provide valuable clues about the patient's condition.
- **Clinical intuition**: With experience, many clinicians develop a kind of 'sixth sense' that guides them in their assessment.

6. Documentation and Communication :
- **Record your observations**: Document your observations during the examination in a detailed and structured manner.
- **Share your findings**: Discuss your observations and assessment with the patient, and with other healthcare professionals if necessary.

Carrying out a clinical examination is as much an art as a science. Every patient is unique, and it is essential to approach the examination with openness, curiosity and respect. In internal medicine, with its vast range of possible pathologies, the clinical examination is all the more crucial, and the ability to link signs and symptoms to an underlying pathology is an invaluable skill.

Technical gestures : Inserting venous lines.

Inserting venous lines is a common procedure in hospitals. These devices are used to administer medicines, fluids and blood products, or to draw blood. They can be used for short stays, such as peripheral venous catheters, or long stays, such as central venous catheters.

1. Introduction: Importance of the venous route
   Drug administration: Some drugs can only be administered intravenously.
   Resuscitation and emergencies: The venous route is essential for the rapid administration of fluids or medication in an emergency.
   Blood sampling : Catheters make it easy to draw blood for analysis.
2. Peripheral venous catheter (PVC) :
   Indications: Short-term treatments, blood sampling.
   Preferred sites: Veins on the back of the hand and forearm.
   Application technique: rigorous disinfection, application with a needle, fixation and permeability check.
   Management and maintenance: Regular monitoring, renewal as required and recommended.
3. Central venous catheters (CVC) :
   Indications: Long-term treatments, parenteral nutrition, chemotherapy, vasoactive drugs, dialysis.

Preferred sites: internal jugular vein, subclavian vein, femoral vein.

Fitting technique: Requires a strict sterile technique, often under radiological or ultrasound control.

Management and maintenance: rigorous monitoring to prevent complications, sterile dressings, dedicated lines for certain infusions.

4. Possible complications :

Thrombophlebitis: inflammation of a vein caused by a blood clot.

Infection: At the puncture site or systemically.

Extravasation: involuntary passage of medication or liquid outside the vein, which may cause tissue damage.

Catheter obstruction: By a clot or precipitated drug.

5. Good Practices :

Rigorous asepsis: hand washing, use of sterile gloves, careful disinfection of the puncture site.

Appropriate technique: Choice of catheter size depending on the treatment, checking venous return.

Patient education: Explain the reason for the procedure and the signs of complications to watch out for.

Withdrawal: When no longer required or in the event of complications, following protocols to minimise risks.

The insertion and management of venous lines are essential skills for internal medicine nurses, given the diversity of patients and treatments administered. Ongoing training and updating of knowledge are crucial to ensure patient safety and effective treatment.

Direct debits.

Blood samples play a crucial role in the diagnostic and therapeutic management of internal medicine patients. They provide precise information about an individual's health, identifying the presence of pathogenic micro-organisms, biochemical anomalies or markers of specific diseases.

1. Introduction: Relevance of sampling
    Diagnostic guidance: Identifying the underlying cause of a pathology or symptom.
    Therapeutic monitoring: monitoring the effectiveness or side effects of a treatment.
    Screening: Identifying a disease at an early stage or determining the risk of developing a certain condition.
2. Types of samples commonly taken in internal medicine :
    Blood :
        Complete blood count
        Biochemical check-up (ionogram, kidney and liver functions, etc.)
        Hormone levels
        Specific markers (e.g. troponin for myocardial infarction)
    Urinary :
        ECBU (Urine CytoBacteriological Examination)
        Biochemical assays
        Search for proteins or other pathological elements
    Bowel movements :
        Coproculture (if infection is suspected)
        Search for occult blood
    Cerebrospinal fluid (CSF): In cases of suspected meningitis or other neurological pathologies.
    Punctures :
        Lumbar puncture

Pleural puncture
Ascites puncture
Biopsies (liver, kidney, etc.)

Pap smear: For example, vaginal smear for cervical cancer screening.

3. Sampling techniques :

Aseptic conditions: To ensure that samples are not contaminated.

Appropriate equipment: Use specific tubes or culture media depending on the type of sample.

Correct technique: Minimise the risk of complications for the patient and ensure the reliability of the sample.

4. Transport and storage :

Packaging: Some samples need to be stored at specific temperatures or protected from light.

Speed: Speed of delivery to the laboratory is often crucial to the reliability of results.

5. Interpretation of results :

Normal vs. Abnormal: Compare results with reference values.

Clinical correlation: Relate the results to the patient's clinical picture.

6. Communication with the laboratory :

Discussions: Talk to the laboratory to understand unexpected results or request additional analyses.

Ongoing training: Analysis methods are evolving, so it's crucial to keep up to date.

Blood sampling is a fundamental tool for healthcare professionals in internal medicine, and its correct performance and interpretation are essential for optimal patient care. Nurses play a central role in this process, from collecting the sample to communicating the results to the patient and the healthcare team.

Administration specific treatments.

The administration of specific treatments is one of the central tasks of the internal medicine nurse. These often complex treatments require a thorough understanding, attention to detail and close collaboration with the medical team.

1. Introduction: The versatility of the nursing role

   Adapting therapy: Every patient is unique. His or her needs, history and response to treatment require constant adaptation.

   Educate and reassure: The nurse informs the patient about his or her therapy, explains the potential benefits and risks, and ensures that the patient and his or her family understand the treatment plan.
2. Common treatments in internal medicine :

   Antibiotics: Whether intravenous, oral or injected, they are frequently used to treat various infections.

   Corticosteroids: Used in inflammatory or auto-immune diseases.

   Anticoagulants: Prevention and treatment of thrombosis.

   Immunosuppressants: used in particular for autoimmune diseases or after transplants.

   Chemotherapy : For the treatment of certain cancers or haematological diseases.

   Substitute treatments: such as insulin for diabetes or thyroid hormones.
3. Administration techniques :

   Oral: tablets, capsules, syrups.

   Injection: Intravenous, intramuscular, subcutaneous.

   Perfusion: Over variable durations, requires close monitoring.

   Topical: creams, gels, patches.

   Inhalation: Sprays, aerosols, nebulisations.

4. Monitoring and side effects :
- **Clinical monitoring**: Observe for the appearance of adverse symptoms or signs of improvement.
- **Biological tests**: Some treatments require regular monitoring of blood parameters.
- **Managing side-effects**: Recognising, treating and, if necessary, adapting treatment in the event of an undesirable effect.

5. Therapeutic education :
- **Clear explanations**: Helping patients to understand their illness and treatment.
- **Adherence to treatment** : Discuss potential barriers and encourage regular uptake.
- **Self-administration**: Teaching patients how to administer their own treatment if necessary (e.g. insulin injections).

6. Coordination with the care team :
- **Targeted communications**: Sharing observations and any treatment-related problems with doctors.
- **Multidisciplinary collaboration**: working with pharmacists, physiotherapists, dieticians, etc.

The administration of specific treatments is a heavy responsibility that rests on the shoulders of the internal medicine nurse. It requires not only technical skills, but also the ability to communicate, educate and adapt to each patient. In this context, the nurse plays a pivotal role, guaranteeing patient safety while optimising therapeutic effectiveness.

Chapter 4:
INTERPROFESSIONAL COLLABORATION

Working with the internist:
communication and rapport.

Working closely with the internist is an essential part of the nursing profession. This collaboration involves clear, precise and respectful communication, to ensure optimal patient care. The nurse-internist relationship is all the more crucial in internal medicine, a complex speciality concerned with multi-system pathologies.

1. Understanding the role of the internist :
     Medical expertise: internists are experts in internal pathologies, which are often chronic and multi-systemic.
     Therapeutic decisions: He makes decisions concerning treatment and diagnostic orientations.
2. The importance of communication :
     Passing on information: Nurses are in the front line when it comes to observing the patient's progress. Transmitting this information accurately is essential.
     Two-way exchange: If the nurse transmits information to the doctor, the latter must also communicate his decisions and reasoning to the nurse.
     Multi-disciplinary meetings: These are opportunities to discuss complex cases and define a collective therapeutic strategy.
3. The day-to-day relationship :
     Mutual respect: Recognising the expertise of others, valuing their role and skills.

Collaboration: working hand in hand, particularly in emergency situations or when complex decisions have to be made.

Continuing education: The internist can play a formative role for the nurse, helping him or her to better understand certain pathologies or treatments.

4. Managing disagreements :

Dialogue: In the event of a difference of opinion, it is essential to establish a constructive dialogue, putting the patient's interests first.

Feedback: Feedback is essential to improve collaboration. It is important to be able to discuss what is working well and where improvements can be made.

5. Communication with the patient :

Coordinated approach: The nurse and doctor must present a coherent vision and information to the patient, even if each brings their own perspective.

Role of translator: The nurse can sometimes act as an intermediary, explaining to the patient, in simpler words, what the doctor has prescribed or diagnosed.

6. Evolution of the relationship :

From hierarchy to collaboration: While in the past the relationship was often perceived as hierarchical, today the emphasis is on horizontal collaboration, where each healthcare professional contributes his or her unique expertise.

Interdependence: Optimal patient care requires the synergy of the entire care team.

Collaboration between the nurse and the internist is a delicate but essential dance. It requires trust, open communication and mutual respect. In internal medicine, where cases can be complex, this collaboration is the key to successful management and constant improvement in the quality of care.

Shared decision-making.

Shared decision making (SDM) is a collaborative process in which the healthcare professional and the patient work together to make a medical decision. This approach emphasises partnership, respect for the patient's values and preferences, and the use of the best available evidence. In internal medicine, given the complexity of cases, PDP is particularly relevant.

1. Foundations of shared decision-making :
   Respect for individual values: Each patient has his or her own values, concerns and aspirations. PDP respects these essential elements.
   Right to autonomy: Patients have the right to actively participate in their own care and to make decisions about their health.
2. The PDP process :
   Patient information: Providing patients with clear, precise and comprehensible information about the options available, and their advantages and disadvantages.
   Active listening: Understanding the patient's preferences, values and concerns.
   Discussion: Openly discuss the different options, weighing up their advantages and disadvantages against the patient's expectations and concerns.
   Joint decision-making: The healthcare professional and the patient agree on the best decision to take.
3. The benefits of PDP :
   Personalised care: Treatment is tailored to the patient's needs and preferences.
   Better adherence to treatment: Patients are more likely to follow a course of treatment when they have been involved in the decision.
   Increased satisfaction: Patients feel valued, listened to and involved.

4. The challenges of PDP :
  Time: PDP can take longer than traditional decision-making approaches.
  Training: Healthcare professionals need to be trained in this approach to be effective.
  Limitations of evidence: Not all medical decisions are supported by solid evidence, which can complicate PDP.
5. PDP in internal medicine :
  Complexity of cases: Internal medicine patients may present with multiple and complex pathologies, requiring a nuanced approach.
  Multidisciplinary team: Decision-making may involve several specialists, emphasising the importance of communication and coordination.
  Ethical challenges: Internal medicine can sometimes present ethical dilemmas, where PDP plays a crucial role in ensuring that the patient is at the heart of decisions.

Shared decision-making represents a major change in the way healthcare is delivered. It values the experience and expertise of the patient, while drawing on the clinical skills of the healthcare professional. In internal medicine, it means navigating the complexity of cases with the patient as a full partner.

Working together
with other departments: Medical imaging.

Medical imaging plays a crucial role in internal medicine. It is used not only to make a diagnosis, but also to monitor the progress of a pathology, guide certain interventions and contribute to medical research. The interaction between nurses and the world of imaging is essential to guarantee quality care.

1. Imaging modalities in internal medicine :
   Radiography: One of the oldest forms of imaging, it uses X-rays to visualise bones and certain tissues.

   Ultrasound: Uses sound waves to produce images, commonly used to examine the heart, vessels, liver and other organs.

   Computed tomography (CT): An advanced form of radiography that produces cross-sectional images of the body.

   Magnetic resonance imaging (MRI): uses powerful magnets and radio waves to produce detailed images.

   Scintigraphy: Uses radioactive substances to assess the function of certain organs.
2. The role of the nurse in medical imaging :
   Preparing the patient: Explain the procedure, check medical history, administer contrast agents if necessary.

   Post-examination follow-up: Monitor any reactions to the contrast agents and ensure that the patient is feeling well after the examination.

   Communication: acting as a link between the patient, the radiologist and the internist, in particular by passing on important information or patient concerns.
3. The diagnostic importance of imaging :
   Detection: pinpointing an anomaly or disease at an early stage.

   Localisation: to pinpoint the location of a lesion or tumour.

   Characterisation: differentiating a benign mass from a malignant one, or determining the nature of an anomaly.
4. Interventional imaging :
   Guided biopsies : Tissue sampling for analysis using an imaging modality.

Catheterisation: using images to guide the introduction of a catheter into the body.
5. Challenges and concerns :
Radiation protection: Minimising radiation exposure for patients and medical staff.
Allergies and interactions: Some contrast agents can cause reactions.
Quality and interpretation: Ensuring optimum image quality and accurate interpretation of results.
6. Innovations and the future of medical imaging :
Advanced technologies: Development of new modalities and improvement of existing techniques to obtain better quality images with less risk.
Artificial intelligence: Using AI to improve image detection and interpretation.

Medical imaging is a cornerstone of internal medicine. Close collaboration between nurses, radiology technologists and doctors is essential to ensure quality care and informed decision-making. Technology is evolving rapidly, offering exciting opportunities to further improve diagnosis and treatment in internal medicine.

Surgery.

Surgery, although generally associated with distinct surgical specialities, interacts closely with internal medicine. Indeed, many internal medicine patients may require surgery or are in the post-operative phase. For the internal medicine nurse, understanding the surgical aspects is fundamental to ensuring optimal care.

1. The interaction between internal medicine and surgery :
Pre-operative consultations: assessment of patients by the internist prior to surgery to detect underlying

medical problems or optimise pre-operative conditions.

Post-operative monitoring: Monitoring of potential medical complications following surgery.

2. The nurse's role in surgery :

Pre-operative preparation: patient education, medical history, skin preparation, verification of pre-operative tests and coordination with the surgical team.

Post-operative care: monitoring vital signs, pain management, wound care, early mobilisation of the patient and early detection of complications.

Communication: acting as a link between the patient, the surgical team and the internist.

3. Post-operative complications :

Cardiovascular complications: heart attack, arrhythmia, heart failure.

Respiratory complications: Pneumonia, atelectasis, pulmonary embolism.

Renal complications: acute renal failure, urinary tract infections.

Infectious complications: surgical site infections, septicaemia.

4. Surgery and multi-pathological patients :

Risk assessment: Patients with multiple co-morbidities may present increased risks during surgery.

Pre-operative optimisation: medication management, stabilisation of chronic illnesses and physical preparation.

5. Specific challenges in internal medicine :

Unscheduled surgery: managing surgical emergencies for patients already hospitalised for medical reasons.

Informed consent: Ensuring that the patient understands the risks and benefits of the procedure, particularly if he or she has cognitive impairment or other complex medical problems.

6. The importance of collaboration :

Multidisciplinary team: Close collaboration between nurses, surgeons, anaesthetists and internists to ensure comprehensive care.

Multidisciplinary consultation meetings: Discussion of complex cases to determine the best surgical and medical approach.

Surgery is a crucial part of the care pathway for many internal medicine patients. For nurses, an in-depth knowledge of the surgical implications and close collaboration with the surgical team are essential to ensure holistic and optimal patient care.

Palliative care.

Palliative care plays an essential role in internal medicine. It aims to improve the quality of life of patients and their families in the face of the consequences of a potentially fatal illness, by relieving pain and physical, psychological and spiritual suffering. For internal medicine nurses, mastery of the principles of palliative care is crucial.

1. Understanding palliative care :

Definition and principles : Discussing the philosophy of palliative care and how it differs from curative care.

The aims of palliative care: pain relief, psychological support, spirituality, maintaining dignity and informed decision-making.

2. The palliative care nurse :

Holistic assessment: understanding the patient as a whole, including physiological, psychological, social and spiritual aspects.

Management of pain and other symptoms: pharmacological and non-pharmacological techniques for the relief of pain, dyspnoea, anxiety and other symptoms.

Psychological and spiritual support: listening, offering comfort, facilitating discussions about the end of life.

3. Communication in palliative care :

Discussions on care objectives: Raising the patient's wishes and preferences, anticipating medical decisions at the end of life.

The gentle truth: How to talk about the end of life without taking away hope.

Communication with the family: integrating the family into the care process, offering support and information.

4. Ethical challenges :

Therapeutic overkill vs. letting go: Finding the balance between continuing treatment and accepting the end of life.

Advance directives: the importance and role of directives concerning medical decisions at the end of life.

Euthanasia and assisted suicide: Addressing the debates and ethical implications in different cultural and legal contexts.

5. Support for the care team :

Compassion fatigue: Recognising and managing the emotional exhaustion associated with palliative care.

Supervision and self-care: the importance of reflection, peer support and self-preservation strategies.

Training and resources: Opportunities to improve skills and knowledge in palliative care.

6. The evolution of palliative care :

Palliative care at home: The challenges and benefits of caring for patients outside a hospital setting.

Technology and palliative care: How innovations can support palliative care.

Research and development: New approaches, studies and protocols to improve palliative care.

In internal medicine, palliative care is invaluable in supporting patients in the advanced stages of their illness. The nurse, as the linchpin of the care team, plays a central role in ensuring that these patients enjoy the best possible quality of life at their most vulnerable moments.

Chapter 5:
EMOTIONAL CHALLENGES AND PSYCHOLOGICAL SUPPORT

Managing stress and burnout.

Managing stress and burnout is a fundamental issue in the medical field, particularly in internal medicine where the intensity of care can be increased. Nurses, on the front line, are particularly exposed. A proactive approach is essential if they are to provide optimum patient care while preserving their own well-being.

1. Recognising the signs of stress and burnout :
   - **Physical symptoms**: Chronic fatigue, headaches, insomnia, muscle pain.
   - **Emotional symptoms**: Irritability, feeling overwhelmed, anxiety, depression.
   - **Behavioural symptoms**: Social withdrawal, reduced performance, task avoidance.
2. Understanding the causes :
   - **Workload**: Long and irregular working hours, multiple responsibilities, lack of resources.
   - **Team dynamics**: interpersonal conflicts, lack of support, communication problems.
   - **Emotional factors** : Intense ties with patients, frequent confrontations with suffering and death.
3. Stress management strategies :
   - **Relaxation techniques**: deep breathing, meditation, yoga.
   - **Time management**: prioritising tasks, taking regular breaks, delegating where possible.
   - **Professional limits**: knowing how to say no, recognising your limits, asking for help.

4. Preventing burnout :

Work-life balance: Valuing time away from work, disconnecting, having hobbies.

Professional support: supervision, discussion groups, stress management training.

Regular assessment: self-assessment, peer feedback, follow-up with a mental health professional if necessary.

5. Cultivating resilience :

Personal reflection: Understand your own stress triggers, recognise your strengths and limitations.

Develop a support network: confidants, mentors, peer group.

Continuing training: Reinforce your skills, learn new methods for managing stress.

6. The importance of institutional support :

Well-being programmes: Establishment initiatives for mental health, support groups.

Prevention policies: Recognition of and action against burnout as an organisational problem.

Training opportunities: Workshops, seminars and training to manage stress and prevent burnout.

7. External resources :

Therapy: Finding a space to discuss professional and personal challenges.

Coaching and mentoring: Benefit from the advice and experience of other professionals.

Professional associations: resources, workshops and support communities.

In an environment as demanding as internal medicine, nurses need to arm themselves with strategies and resources to navigate through the daily challenges. Proactive stress management and the prevention of burnout are essential not only for the well-being of the nurse, but also to ensure optimal patient care.

The importance of empathy and communication.

Empathy and communication are essential pillars in the medical world, and particularly so for internal medicine nurses. Navigating at the heart of ailments and emotions, the nurse is often the first point of contact, the link between the patient and the rest of the medical team. In this dynamic, the ability to understand, feel and communicate becomes crucial.

Empathy is the ability to put yourself in another person's shoes, to perceive their feelings, to enter their world without judgement. In internal medicine, where pathologies are diverse and often complex, and where patients are sometimes overwhelmed by an avalanche of information and treatments, the nurse's empathy makes all the difference. It soothes and reassures. It builds a bond of trust, making the patient a player in his or her own recovery.

But empathy alone is not enough. It must be accompanied by clear, precise and appropriate communication. Every patient is unique, with his or her own experience, culture and fears. Adapting what you say, choosing the right words, avoids misunderstandings, reassures and educates. When nurses take the time to explain a treatment, answer a question or explain a procedure in detail, they are giving patients the tools they need to understand their situation, cooperate and move forward.

This alliance between empathy and communication also shapes the relationship with those close to the patient. In the corridors of internal medicine, family and friends all gravitate, worried, hoping for news, seeking to understand. The nurse's empathy can allay their fears, and his or her communication can light their way.

But this delicate dance between empathy and communication doesn't stop there. It extends to the medical team. Understanding a colleague's needs, anticipating a request, clearly communicating an observation - all this facilitates teamwork, making care smoother and more efficient.

Finally, beyond the tangible benefits, empathy and communication enrich nurses themselves. They enable them to forge deep bonds, find meaning in their work and get through difficult days. They remind them that behind every medical file there is a human being, with his or her hopes, fears and dreams. And that every interaction, every word, every gesture counts. In internal medicine, as elsewhere, empathy and communication are not just skills, they are the very essence of care.

Managing difficult cases : Patients at the end of life.

Patients at the end of life are a particularly emotional and complex area of internal medicine. Accompanying these people in their final moments requires not only clinical expertise, but also a depth of humanity. This is a time when quality of life, dignity and respect for the patient's wishes are paramount.

When a patient enters this end-of-life phase, everything changes. Therapeutic objectives shift from a curative to a palliative approach. The emphasis is no longer on cure, but on pain relief, comfort, well-being and psychological support. It's about understanding and accepting that sometimes not doing something is just as important as doing it, and that relentless treatment is not always in the patient's best interests.

But this period is also marked by a series of emotional and ethical challenges. Nurses in internal medicine are often faced with difficult decisions. When should treatment be stopped? How do you approach discussions about resuscitation, nutrition or artificial hydration? How do you respect the patient's wishes while taking account of medical recommendations and the feelings of the family? These dilemmas require careful listening, clear communication and, above all, a great deal of empathy.

Accompanying a patient at the end of life also means witnessing intense moments. Tearful goodbyes, regrets, reconciliations, moments of grace when life and death come together in a silent dance. It is at these moments that the nurse plays an essential role, not only as a healthcare professional, but also as a human being. Being there, offering a hand to shake, a smile, a comforting word, can make all the difference.

It is also crucial to support the family and loved ones. They are going through a period of grief, confusion and anxiety. By guiding them, informing them, listening to them and comforting them, we can help them get through this delicate period, mourn and find meaning in their loss.

However, it is important to recognise the emotional impact on nurses themselves. Regularly caring for patients at the end of life can lead to burnout and even vicarious trauma. It is therefore essential to take care of oneself, seek support, recognise one's own emotions and respond to them with kindness.

End-of-life care is a reminder of the very essence of internal medicine: caring for human beings in all their complexity, with compassion and dignity. It's a powerful reminder of the fragility of life, but also of the beauty and depth of human bonds.

The bad news.

Talking about bad news in the medical context is like plunging into the heart of one of the profession's most delicate challenges. Whether it's an unexpected diagnosis, an unfavourable prognosis or a medical complication, breaking difficult news is an arduous task that requires tact, compassion and skill.

The first impact of bad news is shock. The words can seem to float through the air, heavy with meaning, creating a shockwave that numbs the minds of the patient and their loved ones. For the nurse or doctor, it's an often-repeated reality, but for the person receiving the news, it's a singular, shattering moment that divides life into a before and an after.

Breaking bad news therefore requires careful preparation. It is essential to choose the right time and place, to guarantee confidentiality and to ensure that the patient is accompanied if possible. The tone, the words chosen and the clarity of the information all count. The healthcare professional must strive to be both factual and empathetic, avoiding medical jargon while being honest and transparent.

Communication involves more than simply passing on information. It involves actively listening, perceiving the patient's emotions, answering their questions and allaying their concerns. It's an exchange, a dialogue, where emotional support is as important as the information itself.

Reactions to bad news are many and varied. Some patients may go into shock, others may cry, some may ask lots of questions while others may want to be left alone. Recognising and respecting these reactions is crucial. Nurses must be ready to offer support, refer to additional resources if necessary, or simply be there, offering a shoulder to lean on.

It is also essential to involve the family and close friends. They play a crucial role in the emotional support of the patient and must be informed, with the patient's consent, so that they can best accompany their loved one through this ordeal.

But beyond the patient, breaking bad news also has an impact on the healthcare professional. If left unmanaged, this emotional burden can lead to burnout, feelings of guilt or sadness. It is therefore vital for nurses to take care of themselves, seeking support from colleagues, supervision or continuing education.

Breaking bad news means navigating the murky waters of human emotions, seeking to bring clarity, support and compassion to one of life's most difficult moments. It's a powerful reminder of the importance of humanity in medical practice.

Chapter 6:
PROCEDURES AND PROTOCOLS SPECIFIC TO INTERNAL MEDICINE

Isolation and hygiene protocols.

Isolation and hygiene protocols are an integral part of hospital routine, and are of paramount importance in ensuring the safety of patients, nursing staff and visitors. These preventive measures serve not only to prevent the spread of nosocomial infections, but also to protect vulnerable patients with weakened immune systems.

By its very nature, the hospital is a place where many germs, bacteria and viruses coexist. Some patients are admitted with infectious diseases, while others may be at risk of contracting them because of their state of health. In this context, hygiene and isolation take on their full importance.

Hygiene protocols encompass a range of practices. Hand washing is the first and most fundamental measure. It has been proven that effective and regular hand washing considerably reduces the risk of transmission. It is therefore crucial that every member of medical staff, from doctors to nurses to care assistants, adheres strictly to this protocol.
Other hygiene measures include regular cleaning and disinfection of surfaces, particularly in high-risk areas such as operating theatres or intensive care units. Medical equipment, from simple stethoscopes to complex machines, must also be regularly cleaned and disinfected.

Isolation protocols are put in place when a patient is known or suspected to be a carrier of a contagious infection. Depending on the type of infection, different levels of isolation may be necessary:

> **Contact isolation:** for diseases transmitted by direct contact, such as certain strains of resistant bacteria. Care staff must wear gloves and gowns when they come into contact with patients.

> **Respiratory isolation:** for airborne diseases such as tuberculosis. A mask is required to enter the patient's room.

> **Protective isolation:** for patients with a severely weakened immune system, such as after a bone marrow transplant. The aim is to protect the patient from external infections.

These protocols can sometimes seem restrictive, and it is true that being in isolation can be a lonely and difficult experience for the patient. But it is vital to remember that these measures are put in place to protect everyone: the patient, the nursing staff and other patients.

Strict adherence to these protocols requires ongoing training, awareness and vigilance. Nurses play a central role here, not only by ensuring that these measures are applied, but also by educating patients, their families and even their colleagues about their importance.

Ultimately, isolation and hygiene protocols are an expression of the fundamental promise of medicine: "Primum non nocere", or "First, do no harm". In a constantly changing medical world, where germs and bacteria are evolving and becoming increasingly resistant, this promise is more important than ever.

Management of internal emergencies: decompensation, shock, etc.

In the context of internal medicine, nurses are often on the front line in identifying and responding to emergency situations. Confronted with a multitude of pathologies and patient profiles, they must be prepared to manage sudden crises, decompensations or states of shock. These situations require rapid action, clinical expertise and effective communication.

1. Early recognition :
Before an emergency occurs, observation is key. Nurses must be able to detect subtle signs of deterioration in a patient. Changes in vital signs, consciousness, breathing or complexion can be indicators of an impending emergency. Ongoing training and experience play a crucial role in developing this observation skill.

2. Decompensation :
Decompensation is an exacerbation or worsening of a chronic illness. For example, cardiac decompensation may manifest itself as sudden shortness of breath, rapid weight gain due to fluid retention or increased fatigue. The nurse must recognise these signs, initiate the prescribed treatment, such as the administration of diuretics, and quickly inform the medical team.

3. Shock states :
Shock is a medical emergency situation characterised by insufficient perfusion of the organs. It can have different origins: haemorrhagic, cardiogenic, septic, etc. Nurses must be able to identify the type of shock, provide appropriate first aid, such as setting up a venous access line and administering solutions, and alert the medical team.

4. Communication :
In any emergency situation, clear and concise communication is essential. Nurses must be able to pass

on relevant information quickly to doctors, other nurses and, where appropriate, the patient's family. This communication must be factual, focusing on vital signs, observed symptoms, interventions carried out and the patient's response.

5. Teamwork :

A medical emergency is a team effort. Every member of the team, from the doctor to the nurse to the orderly, has a role to play. Effective coordination, respect for roles and mutual trust are essential for optimum patient care.

6. Post-crisis :

Once the situation has stabilised, the nurse's work does not stop. They must monitor the patient to detect any complications, ensure that all treatments are administered and that the doctors are kept informed of the patient's progress. In addition, a debriefing may be necessary to analyse the situation, discuss what went well and identify areas for improvement.

Emergency management in internal medicine is a test of nurses' skill, judgement and resilience. But with the right training, practical experience and the support of a strong team, they are well equipped to meet these challenges and deliver the highest quality care to their patients.

Monitoring chronic patients.

Monitoring chronic patients is a major aspect of internal medicine. The management of chronic diseases such as diabetes, hypertension and lung disease requires a comprehensive, patient-centred approach, combining clinical expertise, therapeutic education and long-term support. Nurses play a central role in this context.

1. Understanding the disease :
Before they can provide effective support to a patient, nurses need to have an in-depth knowledge of the disease in question. This includes its pathophysiology, common symptoms, potential complications and recommended treatments.

2. Therapeutic education :
One of the nurses' key roles is to educate patients about their illness and its treatment. This may include information on taking medication, recognising the signs of decompensation, or the importance of a suitable diet and lifestyle. The aim is to make patients autonomous and active participants in their own care.

3. Regular monitoring :
Regular monitoring means that any deterioration in health or complications can be identified at an early stage. At these appointments, the nurse assesses the effectiveness of the treatment, the occurrence of side effects and ensures that the patient understands and adheres to the prescribed treatment.

4. Care coordination :
Often, the chronic patient is followed by several specialists. Nurses can play a central role in coordinating this care, ensuring fluid communication between the various health professionals and ensuring continuity of care.

5. Psychological support :
Living with a chronic illness can be a source of anxiety, frustration or depression for patients. Nurses are often the patient's first point of contact, and as such it is essential that they are able to offer psychological support, listening to patients' concerns and referring them to a specialist professional if necessary.

6. Health promotion :
In addition to drug treatment, the approach to chronic illness often involves lifestyle changes. Whether it's encouraging physical activity, dietary advice or stopping smoking, nurses play an active role in health promotion.

7. Therapeutic adherence :

One of the greatest challenges in the management of chronic diseases is to ensure that patients continue to adhere to their treatment. Nurses, through their regular contact with patients, are at the forefront of identifying obstacles to adherence and working with patients to overcome them.

Monitoring chronic patients is a long-term task, requiring patience, empathy and clinical expertise. But it also offers nurses the opportunity to build lasting relationships with their patients, and to support them throughout their care pathway, with the ultimate reward of improving their quality of life.

Chapter 7:
TOOLS AND TECHNOLOGY
IN INTERNAL MEDICINE

The evolution
electronic medical records.

The evolution of electronic medical records (EMRs) has dramatically transformed the way healthcare is delivered, documented and managed. These digital systems have replaced traditional paper records, ushering in an era of medical accuracy, efficiency and interoperability.

1. From the origins to the digital age :
Initially, medical records were simply handwritten notes, often scattered between different providers and hospitals. The need for centralisation and better organisation led to the gradual adoption of EMRs, beginning in the 1960s and 1970s, but their use became widespread in the early 21st century.

2. Advantages of EMRs :
EMRs have brought a series of tangible benefits. They have improved efficiency by reducing the need to repeatedly enter identical information, promoted better coordination of care between different providers, and minimised medical errors thanks to the legibility and availability of information.

3. Integration and interoperability :
As technology has advanced, EMRs have evolved to integrate with other systems, such as pharmaceutical databases, laboratories or medical imaging systems. This interoperability has made it easier to communicate and

share data between different institutions and medical specialities.

4. Advanced features :
Over time, EMRs have incorporated increasingly advanced functionalities, such as the detection of drug interactions, reminders for prevention or patient monitoring, and analysis tools to improve the quality of care.

5. Challenges and concerns :
Despite their many advantages, EMRs are not without their challenges. Concerns about privacy and data security, difficulties with interoperability between different systems, and the need for ongoing training for healthcare staff have all been raised.

6. The future of DME :
With the rise of artificial intelligence and telemedicine, EMRs are set to become even more sophisticated. They could incorporate predictive analysis tools, enable real-time monitoring of patients or adapt to virtual consultations.

7. The impact on the role of carers :
The move to digital technology has required healthcare professionals to adapt. While some mentioned a feeling of distance from the patient because of the digital interface, others emphasised the opportunities offered by these tools to improve the quality of care.

The development of electronic medical records has redefined modern medical practice. Although they present certain challenges, their potential for improving care, coordination and prevention is undeniable. As technology advances, EMRs are likely to continue to evolve and adapt to the changing needs of the medical field.

Use of specific medical equipment: monitors, pumps, etc.

The use of specific medical devices is a fundamental aspect of modern medicine. This equipment, ranging from monitors to pumps, plays a crucial role in monitoring, diagnosing and treating patients. In the context of internal medicine, mastery of this equipment is essential for nurses.

1. Medical monitors :

Vital signs monitors: These monitor essential parameters such as blood pressure, pulse, oxygen saturation and temperature, either continuously or at regular intervals. These monitors allow rapid detection of variations and anomalies.

Electrocardiograms (ECG): These record the heart's electrical activity, which is essential for detecting arrhythmias or other cardiac abnormalities.

Capnograph monitors: These measure the level of carbon dioxide exhaled, which is particularly useful during sedation or anaesthesia.

2. Pumps and infusions :

Infusion pumps: These are used for the controlled and precise delivery of drugs or solutions. Controlling their operation is essential to avoid over- or under-dosing.

Enteral nutrition pumps: These deliver food directly into the stomach or intestine for patients who are unable to eat orally.

Insulin pumps: For diabetic patients, these pumps deliver a precise amount of insulin, tailored to the patient's needs.

3. Breathing equipment :

Oxygen therapy: Devices such as nasal cannula or oxygen masks are used to administer oxygen to patients in need.

Ventilators: For patients unable to breathe on their own or requiring respiratory support.
4. Diagnostic equipment :
Spirometers: These measure lung capacity and are essential for diagnosing conditions such as asthma or COPD.
Tensiometers: Used to measure blood pressure, a crucial indicator of cardiovascular health.
5. Other commonly used equipment :
Defibrillators: Essential in the event of cardiac arrest, they deliver an electric shock to try to restore a normal heart rhythm.
Medical aspirators: Used to remove secretions or other fluids from the respiratory tract.
Pulsometers: These measure heart rate and oxygen saturation.

It is essential for internal medicine nurses to master this equipment. Each piece of equipment requires specific training, both for use and maintenance. Nurses must also be able to interpret the data provided by these devices, act quickly in the event of an anomaly and communicate effectively with the medical team.
In today's technological age, medical equipment continues to evolve, becoming more precise and more functional. Nurses therefore need to keep abreast of innovations on a regular basis, in order to guarantee optimum, safe patient care.

Telemedicine and its growing role.

Telemedicine is a form of medicine that uses information and communication technologies to provide medical care at a distance. In recent years, telemedicine has grown exponentially, driven by technological advances and the changing needs of society. It is now a fundamental part of the modern medical landscape.

1. Origins of telemedicine :
The first forms of telemedicine appeared with the invention of the telephone. Doctors were able to offer consultations at a distance. With the emergence of the Internet and videoconferencing technologies, the possibilities have expanded considerably.

2. Benefits of telemedicine :
> **Access to care:** This enables patients who are far away or have reduced mobility to access specialist care without having to travel.
> **Lower costs:** fewer journeys, fewer hospital admissions and faster response times can lead to significant savings.
> **Continuity of care:** Telemonitoring enables chronic patients to be monitored continuously and treatments to be adjusted in real time.

3. Telemedicine procedures :
> **Teleconsultation:** Patient and doctor interact in real time via videoconferencing.
> **Telemonitoring:** Remote monitoring of a patient's vital signs and other medical parameters.
> **Tele-expertise:** A doctor seeks the opinion of a specialist colleague on a particular case.

4. The role of nurses :
Nurses play a central role in the implementation of telemedicine, particularly in remote monitoring. They train patients to use the equipment, interpret the data collected and alert doctors to any problems.

5. Challenges and ethical considerations :
> **Confidentiality:** Ensuring the security and confidentiality of data is paramount.
> **Training:** Medical staff must be trained in the use of telemedicine tools.

Doctor-patient relationship: Maintaining a relationship of trust despite the physical distance.

6. Future prospects :

With the development of artificial intelligence and the Internet of Things, telemedicine is set to diversify and intensify. Tools such as connected watches could enable patients to be monitored even more closely.

Telemedicine is redefining the way in which medical care is delivered. It offers new opportunities, but also new challenges. In this rapidly changing context, the role of nurses as intermediaries between technology and patients is more crucial than ever.

Chapter 8:
PREVENTION AND PUBLIC HEALTH

The importance of vaccination.

Vaccination is one of the most important and effective medical advances in modern history. It has prevented countless deaths and reduced the prevalence of many infectious diseases that used to wreak havoc. Exploring the importance of vaccination requires a thorough understanding of its benefits, both for the individual and for society.

1. The mechanism of vaccination :
Vaccination involves introducing a weakened, inactivated infectious agent, or part of it, into the body in order to stimulate an immune response. The immune system recognises this agent as a threat, develops antibodies to fight it, and then remembers this information. If the person is later exposed to the actual disease, their immune system is ready to fight it quickly.

2. Personal protection :
- **Disease prevention :** Vaccines protect against many potentially serious and even fatal diseases.
- **Reduced severity:** Even if a vaccinated person contracts the disease, the severity of the infection is generally reduced.
- **Lifelong protection:** Certain vaccines, administered during childhood, can offer protection that lasts a lifetime.

3. Collective immunity :
When a sufficiently high proportion of the population is vaccinated, it becomes difficult for a disease to spread. This protects even those who cannot be vaccinated, such

as people with certain medical contraindications. This overall protection is known as herd immunity.

4. Disease eradication :

Vaccination has made it possible to completely eradicate certain diseases. The most notable case is that of smallpox, which was declared eradicated in 1980 thanks to a worldwide vaccination campaign.

5. Reducing healthcare costs :

Preventing a disease through vaccination is far less expensive than treating it. Vaccination saves huge sums in medical costs and costs associated with lost productivity.

6. Vaccine safety :

Although vaccines undergo rigorous clinical testing before approval, their safety continues to be monitored once they are on the market. Serious side effects are extremely rare.

7. Controversies and myths :

Unfortunately, despite their proven benefits, vaccines are the subject of many misconceptions and mistrust. Sound scientific evidence is crucial to addressing public concerns and ensuring high vaccination coverage.

Vaccination is a powerful medical tool that has transformed public health. It saves lives, protects populations and reduces the burden of infectious diseases. In the current context of globalisation and frequent travel, vaccination remains one of the best defences against potential epidemics.

Disease prevention non-transmissible.

Non-communicable diseases (NCDs) encompass a wide range of conditions that are not caused by direct infection. They include heart disease, stroke, diabetes, cancer and chronic respiratory diseases, among others. Given that NCDs are responsible for the vast majority of deaths worldwide, their prevention is a major public health issue.

The key lies in awareness, education and the adoption of healthy lifestyles.

1. Understanding the underlying causes :
NCDs often have multifactorial origins, but some common causes include poor eating habits, lack of physical activity, smoking, excessive alcohol consumption and exposure to harmful environmental factors.

2. The importance of a balanced diet :
Eating healthily is essential for preventing NCDs. This includes eating fruit and vegetables, limiting saturated and trans fats, reducing salt and sugar intake, and preferring unprocessed foods.

3. Promoting physical activity:
Regular activity reduces the risk of several NCDs, including heart disease, type 2 diabetes and certain cancers. At least 150 minutes of moderate physical activity a week is recommended.

4. Smoking cessation :
Smoking is the main preventable risk factor for NCDs. Smoking cessation programmes and awareness campaigns can help reduce the prevalence of smoking.

5. Moderate alcohol consumption:
Excessive alcohol consumption can increase the risk of heart disease, cirrhosis of the liver and certain cancers. It is therefore essential to promote responsible drinking.

6. Prevention of harmful exposure:
This may include reducing exposure to air pollutants, hazardous chemicals or harmful radiation.

7. Screening and early detection :
Regular medical check-ups and screening can help detect the early signs of NCDs, allowing for early intervention and better disease management.

8. Education and awareness:
It is essential to educate the public about the risks associated with NCDs and to promote healthy lifestyle

choices. Awareness campaigns, educational programmes and access to reliable information play a crucial role.

9. The role of public policy :
Well-designed policies can foster an environment that supports the prevention of NCDs. This may include regulations on tobacco advertising, taxes on sugary drinks or improved infrastructure to encourage physical activity.

10. Community support:
Communities can play a vital role in creating environments that support healthy choices, such as green spaces for exercise, local farmers' markets or smoking cessation programmes.

NCD prevention requires a holistic approach, combining individual, community and political efforts. Increased awareness and the adoption of healthy behaviours can significantly reduce the burden of these diseases on individuals and society.

Health education.

Health education is a process which aims to enable individuals to acquire the knowledge, skills and attitudes necessary to make informed decisions about their health. This includes an understanding of how lifestyle choices, behaviours and the environment affect health, as well as the ability to act proactively to improve and maintain an optimal state of well-being. Health education plays an essential role in promoting healthy living and preventing disease.

1. Foundations of health education :
   Objectives: Health education aims to improve knowledge, change attitudes and positively influence health-related behaviour.

Principles: Based on evidence, it must be adapted to the age, culture and level of education of individuals.

2. Topics covered :
   Nutrition and healthy eating
   Physical activity
   Personal hygiene
   Mental health and emotional well-being
   Addiction prevention (tobacco, alcohol, drugs)
   Reproductive health and sexuality
   Safety and accident prevention

3. Methodologies :
   Participative approach: actively involving participants in the learning process.
   Practical demonstrations: showing specific techniques or skills.
   Group discussions: sharing experiences and ideas.
   Case studies: Analysing real-life situations to learn from them.
   Multimedia: Use videos, applications or educational games to make learning more engaging.

4. The importance of evaluation :
Regular evaluation of the effectiveness of health education programmes is essential to ensure that they meet the needs of participants and achieve their objectives.

5. The challenges of health education :
   Combating misinformation and myths about health.
   Adapting programmes to a wide range of audiences.
   Ensuring that information is accessible to all.

6. Health education in different contexts :
   Schools: Incorporate health education into school curricula.
   Communities: Organise workshops and seminars to raise awareness among the local population.
   Hospitals and clinics: Providing information to patients on managing their health and illnesses.
   Workplaces: Promoting the health and well-being of employees.

7. The evolution of health education :
With the advent of the Internet and social media, access to health information is greater than ever. However, this also presents the risk of misinformation. Health educators therefore need to be at the cutting edge of technology while maintaining a critical, evidence-based approach.
8. The importance of collaboration :
Health education is most effective when it is carried out in collaboration with other players, such as health professionals, educators, political decision-makers and communities.

Health education is a powerful tool for empowering individuals to take control of their health and well-being. It requires a multi-dimensional approach, tailored to the needs of each individual, and must be constantly updated to remain relevant in our rapidly changing world.

Chapter 9:
COMMON PATHOLOGIES
IN INTERNAL MEDICINE

Autoimmune diseases.

Autoimmune diseases are complex conditions in which the immune system, which is normally designed to protect the body from infection and other external threats, turns against itself, attacking healthy tissues and organs. This misuse of the immune system can have devastating consequences, affecting virtually any organ or system in the body.

1. Understanding autoimmunity :
    - **How the immune system works:** Under normal circumstances, the immune system recognises and eliminates pathogens, while tolerating components of the self. In autoimmune diseases, this distinction is blurred.
    - **Antigens vs. self-antigens: While** foreign antigens normally trigger the immune response, self-antigens, which are part of the self, can also become the target.
2. Common types of autoimmune disease :
    - Rheumatoid arthritis: Affects the joints.
    - **Systemic lupus erythematosus:** May affect many organs.
    - **Multiple sclerosis:** Attacks the central nervous system.
    - **Type 1 diabetes:** The destruction of beta cells in the pancreas leads to a lack of insulin.
    - **Celiac disease:** Reaction to gliadin, a component of gluten.
    - Hashimoto's thyroiditis: Affects the thyroid gland.

Sjögren's syndrome: Affects the exocrine glands, particularly those producing tears and saliva.

3. Causes and risk factors :

Genetics: A family history may increase the risk.

Environment: Viral infections, certain medications and other environmental factors can trigger autoimmune diseases in susceptible individuals.

Hormones: Women are more often affected, suggesting a role for sex hormones.

4. Symptoms and diagnosis :

Symptoms vary greatly depending on the disease and the organs affected. However, fatigue, joint pain and inflammation are common.

Diagnosis is based on clinical symptoms, blood tests (for autoantibodies) and sometimes tissue biopsies.

5. Treatment and management :

Immunosuppressants: Drugs that reduce the activity of the immune system.

Symptomatic treatments: such as anti-inflammatories to reduce pain.

Targeted therapies: Medicines that target specific pathways in the immune system.

Therapeutic education: Patients learn how to manage their disease and recognise the signs of a relapse.

6. Research and the future :

Progress is regularly made in understanding these diseases, leading to new treatments and more personalised therapeutic approaches.

Autoimmune diseases are a challenge for healthcare professionals and patients alike. Research and multidisciplinary management are essential to improve the quality of life of those affected and to make progress towards curative solutions.

Metabolic disorders.

Metabolic disorders encompass a wide range of pathologies resulting from abnormalities in metabolism, i.e. the processes by which our body produces, uses or stores energy. These diseases can be hereditary, resulting from a genetic defect, or acquired, as a result of environmental factors, diet or other illnesses.

1. Introduction to metabolisms :

Definition of metabolism: All the chemical reactions that take place within a cell or organism to produce energy and build or break down molecules.

Catabolism vs Anabolism: Catabolism breaks down large molecules to produce energy, while anabolism uses this energy to build complex molecules.

2. Common metabolic disorders :

Diabetes: An abnormality in blood sugar regulation, mainly due to insulin deficiency or resistance.

Hypercholesterolaemia: Excessive concentration of cholesterol in the blood, often linked to diet or genetic factors.

Gout: Accumulation of uric acid in the blood, which can crystallise in the joints.

Hereditary metabolic diseases: For example, phenylketonuria, an inability to metabolise the amino acid phenylalanine.

3. Causes of metabolic disorders :

Genetic factors: Genetic mutations can affect key enzymes, disrupting metabolic pathways.

Environmental factors: diet, lack of exercise, exposure to certain toxic substances.

Drug interactions: Certain drugs can interfere with metabolism.

4. Symptoms and diagnosis :

    Symptoms vary considerably depending on the specific disorder, and can include fatigue, pain, weight gain or loss, skin abnormalities and more.

    Blood, urine and sometimes genetic tests are commonly used to diagnose metabolic disorders.

5. Treatment and management :

    Dietary interventions: Some disorders require a strict diet to avoid certain nutrients.

    Medication: To regulate metabolism, such as oral hypoglycaemics or insulin for diabetes.

    Enzyme therapies: In some cases, it is possible to supply the deficient enzyme.

6. Prevention and education :

    A balanced diet, regular exercise and limiting exposure to toxins can help prevent many metabolic disorders.

    Patients with hereditary metabolic disorders often benefit from therapeutic education to manage their condition.

7. Research and future prospects :

Significant progress has been made in understanding the molecular and genetic basis of metabolic disorders. Gene therapies, biotechnologies and a better understanding of metabolic pathways are opening up exciting avenues for more targeted and effective treatments.

Metabolic disorders are a vast and diverse field of medicine, requiring specific treatment. With the development of research and technology, it is hoped that many metabolic disorders can be better treated, or even cured, in the future.

Infectious and tropical diseases.

Infectious and tropical diseases represent a vast group of pathologies caused by infectious agents such as bacteria, viruses, parasites and fungi. Many tropical diseases are specific to certain regions of the world, generally hot and humid regions. These diseases are often associated with unfavourable socio-economic conditions, hygiene problems and the absence of robust health systems.

1. Introduction to infectious diseases :
   Transmission: The modes of transmission vary: airborne, droplets, water, food, insects, sexual contact, blood.
   The main infectious agents: bacteria, viruses, parasites, fungi.
2. Major tropical diseases :
   Malaria: Transmitted by the bite of infected mosquitoes, characterised by episodes of fever and chills.
   Dengue: Another mosquito-borne disease, causing high fever and muscle and joint pain.
   Yellow fever: A potentially fatal viral disease also transmitted by mosquitoes.
   Sleeping sickness: Caused by parasites transmitted by the tsetse fly.
3. Recent epidemics :
   Ebola: A highly contagious and often fatal virus.
   Zika: This virus is generally benign in adults, but can cause birth defects in the foetus if a pregnant woman is infected.
4. Diagnosis and symptoms :
   Symptoms vary greatly from one disease to another. They may include fever, skin rashes, muscle and joint pain.
   Diagnosis is generally based on blood tests, samples or cultures.

5. Processing :
  Anti-parasitic drugs: For diseases such as malaria.
  Antibiotics: To treat bacterial infections.
  Vaccinations: Some, such as yellow fever, are essential for travel to certain regions.
6. Prevention :
  Protection against mosquitoes (mosquito nets, repellents, appropriate clothing).
  Vaccinations for certain diseases.
  Access to drinking water and good sanitary facilities.
7. Current challenges :
  Drug resistance: For example, some strains of malaria are now resistant to standard treatments.
  Rapid urbanisation: Increases the risk of disease spreading.
  Climate change: This can expand the habitats of vectors such as mosquitoes.

8. Research and future prospects :

New drugs and vaccines are constantly being sought to combat these diseases. Telemedicine and the use of technology to monitor and predict epidemics are also on the increase.

Infectious and tropical diseases continue to be a major challenge for global health, particularly in resource-limited regions. A combination of research, education, prevention and improved infrastructures is essential to reduce the impact of these diseases.

Chapter 10:
HOLISTIC APPROACHES
AND COMPLEMENTARY

Alternative therapies in internal medicine.

Alternative therapies, also known as complementary and alternative medicine (CAM), refer to a wide range of practices and treatments that are not part of conventional medicine, but are used as a complement or alternative to it. In internal medicine, these approaches can be used to treat or relieve a variety of symptoms or conditions.

1. Introduction to alternative therapies :
    Definition and differentiation: How do these therapies differ from conventional medicine?
    Benefits and risks: Why do some patients and practitioners turn to these methods?
2. Phytotherapy :
    Use of medicinal plants: For example, St John's wort for mild depression or ginkgo biloba to improve memory.
    Available forms: tinctures, powders, capsules, infusions.
3. Acupuncture :
    Basic principles: Balancing the qi or vital energy through specific points on the body.
    Applications: Treatment of pain, headaches, high blood pressure.
4. Homeopathy :
    Like cures like" theory: Using substances that cause symptoms in a healthy individual to treat the same symptoms in a patient.

Dilution and potentiation: Remedies are often extremely diluted.

5. Chiropractic :

Focus on the spine: Manual adjustments to treat musculoskeletal problems.

Applications : Back pain, headaches, joint pain.

6. Meditation and relaxation techniques :

Mindfulness meditation, yoga, tai chi: to reduce stress and improve general well-being.

Applications: Hypertension, mood disorders, sleep disorders.

7. Nutritional approaches :

Specific diets: For example, the Mediterranean diet for heart health or anti-inflammatory diets.

Supplements : Vitamins, minerals, essential fatty acids.

8. Integration of alternative therapies :

Holistic approach: taking into account the whole patient: physical, emotional and social.

Communication with doctors: discussing the benefits and risks of these therapies, ensuring that they do not interfere with conventional treatments.

9. Research and evidence :

Level of evidence: While some therapies have been extensively studied, others lack solid evidence.

Criticism and controversy: Scepticism about the efficacy and safety of certain therapies.

Although alternative therapies offer additional options for patient management, it is essential that these methods are used judiciously, as a complement to conventional medical care, and after consulting a healthcare professional.

The importance of nutrition.

Nutrition, as the science of food and its impact on health, plays a central role in maintaining our well-being, preventing many diseases and helping us to heal. In the field of internal medicine, understanding nutrition is crucial, as it directly influences the course of many pathological conditions.

The essence of nutrition :
Nutrition is not just the act of eating, but rather providing our body with the essential elements (nutrients) it needs to function properly. This includes proteins, carbohydrates, fats, vitamins, minerals and water.
1. Nutrition and prevention :
   Cardiovascular disease: A balanced diet rich in fruit, vegetables and omega-3 fatty acids can reduce the risk of heart disease.
   Diabetes: Maintaining a balanced diet helps to regulate blood sugar levels and prevent type 2 diabetes.
   Osteoporosis: A diet rich in calcium and vitamin D is essential for bone health.
2. Nutrition and the immune system :
Nutrition plays a key role in strengthening the immune system. Micronutrients such as vitamins C and E, zinc and antioxidants are essential for optimal immunity.
3. Weight and metabolism :
   Obesity: An unbalanced diet, rich in sugars and saturated fats, is a major cause of obesity.
   Metabolic disorders: Nutritional imbalances can lead to conditions such as hypothyroidism.
4. Nutrition in the healing process :
Recovering patients have specific nutritional needs to support tissue repair, fight infection and regain energy.
5. Malnutrition and deficiencies :
In certain medical conditions, the body cannot absorb

nutrients properly, leading to deficiencies that can worsen the disease.

6. Eating disorders:

Internal medicine also treats eating disorders such as anorexia or bulimia, where nutrition is at the heart of both the problem and the solution.

7. Psychological aspects of nutrition :

Eating is not just a physical matter. Food choices can be influenced by mood, stress and other psychological factors.

8. Drug interactions :

Some drugs can interact with food, affecting their absorption or effectiveness. Understanding these interactions is crucial in internal medicine.

9. Personalised nutrition:

With advances in genetics, medicine is moving towards a more personalised approach, including nutrition based on an individual's genetic profile.

The importance of nutrition in internal medicine is undeniable. It influences the prevention, development, treatment and cure of many diseases. A thorough understanding of nutrition is therefore essential for all healthcare professionals.

Pain management.

Pain management is one of the main concerns in internal medicine, given the considerable impact of pain on a patient's quality of life. Tackling pain requires a comprehensive approach, as it can be multifactorial, combining physiological, psychological and social elements.

1. Understanding pain :
    Definition and types : Differentiate between acute and chronic pain, nociceptive and neuropathic pain.
    Pain mechanisms: how the body perceives, transmits and reacts to pain.
2. Pain assessment :
    Assessment scales: Tools such as the visual analogue scale (VAS) to quantify pain.
    Case history: Gather information on duration, location, type and triggering or mitigating factors.
3. Pharmacological approaches :
    Analgesics: Paracetamol, non-steroidal anti-inflammatory drugs (NSAIDs), opioids.
    Adjuvant medication: Antidepressants, anticonvulsants, muscle relaxants, for certain specific pains.
    Considerations: Weigh the benefits against the risks, especially with drugs such as opioids.
4. Non-pharmacological therapies :
    Physiotherapy: Exercise, ultrasound, manual therapy.
    Cognitive-behavioural therapies: helping patients to change their perception of pain.
    Relaxation techniques: meditation, deep breathing, biofeedback.
    Interventional procedures: nerve blocks, injections, neurostimulation.
5. Chronic pain :
    Complexity: Recognising the psychological, emotional and physical impact.
    Multidisciplinary approaches: Combination of medical, physical and psychological treatments.
6. Pain management in specific populations :
    Elderly patients: Considerations relating to drug metabolism and polypharmacy.
    Patients with chronic illnesses: For example, pain associated with arthritis or cancer.

Children: Age-appropriate assessment and treatment.

7. Challenges of pain management :

Resistance to treatment: Finding solutions when pain does not respond to the usual treatments.

Dependence and overdose: Particularly with opioid use.

Cultural considerations: Respecting and understanding how different cultures perceive and express pain.

8. The future of pain management :

Research: New drugs, techniques and approaches under development.

Telemedicine: remote management, applications and digital tools.

Pain management is a complex and constantly evolving area of internal medicine. Effective management requires a combination of approaches tailored to each patient, taking into account the nature and severity of their pain, as well as their individual needs and preferences.

Chapter 11:
THE WORKING ENVIRONMENT

Safety and accident prevention.

Safety and accident prevention are paramount in the medical context, and particularly in internal medicine. Ensuring a safe environment not only preserves the health and well-being of patients, but also protects medical staff from potential risks.

1. Understanding the risks :
   Nature of risks: Physical, chemical, biological, radiological.
   Sources of risk: medical equipment, electrical devices, infectious agents, drugs, patients themselves.
2. Preventive measures :
   Staff training: Regular courses on safety, gestures and postures, and handling medical devices.
   Strict protocols: Established procedures for every operation, from simple sampling to complex surgery.
3. Physical safety of patients :
   Falls prevention: Furniture layout, non-slip floors, mobility aids.
   Bed safety: Use of barriers, regular supervision, alarms.
4. Safe handling of medicines :
   Storage: Secure cabinets, restricted access.
   Administration: Double-checking, use of automated equipment to avoid overdoses.
5. Medical equipment and safety :
   Maintenance: Regular checks, updates and replacement if necessary.

Use: Specific training for each piece of equipment, compliance with instructions.

6. Infection prevention :

Strict hygiene: washing hands, wearing gloves, masks and goggles.

Isolation: contagious patients in single rooms, specific protocols for highly infectious diseases.

7. Medical waste management :

Sorting: by type of waste (sharp, infectious, chemical).

Disposal: Incineration, specific treatment for certain types of waste.

8. Preventing medical errors :

Communication: Encouraging dialogue between professionals, ensuring that information is passed on.

Medical records: Regularly updated, easy access for nursing staff.

9. Emergency planning :

Scenarios: Identify potential emergency situations (fires, evacuations, attacks).

Responses: Action protocols, team training, regular exercises.

10. Safety culture :

Feedback: Analyse incidents, even minor ones, to learn from them.

Active promotion: Encouraging a proactive attitude to safety, where every member of staff feels responsible.

In internal medicine, as in all medical fields, safety and accident prevention are central. By implementing rigorous protocols, regularly training staff and instilling a culture in which safety is valued, risks can be considerably reduced, to the benefit of all.

The layout of services internal medicine.

The layout of internal medicine departments is essential to ensure optimum patient care and a smooth workflow for the medical team. As well as meeting the complex medical needs of patients, these layouts must encourage collaboration between healthcare professionals, while ensuring the safety and well-being of patients and staff.

1. Reception and assessment area :

Reception area: A warm welcome for patients and their families.

Consultation offices: Well-lit rooms equipped for initial assessments.

2. Patient rooms :

Provision: Ensuring privacy while allowing medical surveillance.

Facilities : Medical beds, monitors, oxygen points and other necessities.

Comfort: Adequate lighting, furniture for visitors, customisation options.

3. Specialist care areas :

Isolation rooms : For contagious or immunocompromised patients.

Intensive care units: For patients requiring increased monitoring.

4. Work areas for staff :

Care stations: Dedicated areas for preparing medicines, keeping records and coordinating care.

Rest rooms: Places where staff can relax and recharge their batteries.

5. Procedure and examination rooms :

State-of-the-art equipment: For a range of procedures, from gastroscopy to lumbar puncture.

Layout: easy access, logical workflow.

6. Training and meeting rooms :
- **Conference rooms:** For training, team meetings and discussions with families.
- **Technology:** audiovisual equipment, whiteboard, internet connection.

7. Hygiene and sterilisation areas :
- **Washrooms:** For hand washing and disinfection.
- **Sterilisation areas:** For medical instruments.

8. Storage space :
- **Pharmacy:** secure storage of medicines.
- **Equipment storage:** Organised storage of medical supplies, consumables and equipment.

9. Waiting areas :
- **Comfort:** Comfortable seats, distractions such as magazines or screens.
- **Information:** Display boards, screens showing patient status or important announcements.

10. Auxiliary installations :
- **Cafeterias and dining areas:** For patients, families and staff.
- **Green spaces or patios:** For an outdoor break, a moment of relaxation.

The design of internal medicine departments needs to be thought through to meet the unique needs of this speciality. It is a balance between creating a healing environment for patients and providing a functional space for staff. By focusing on comfort, safety and efficiency, an internal medicine department can provide quality care while promoting the well-being of all its occupants.

The challenges of patient mobility and ergonomics for staff.

Patient mobility and staff ergonomics are crucial elements in internal medicine, or in any healthcare environment. They influence not only the well-being and safety of patients, but also the comfort, efficiency and long-term health of carers.

Patient mobility:
Mobility plays a key role in recovery. Patients who are bedridden for too long can develop a range of complications, including pressure sores, muscle atrophy and deep vein thrombosis.
1. Challenges :
> **Physical limitations:** Certain illnesses can impair mobility, either through pain, weakness or neurological deficits.
> **Safety:** The risk of falls can discourage staff from encouraging mobility.
> **Lack of equipment:** Equipment such as walkers or wheelchairs may be inadequate or unsuitable.
> **Environment:** A restricted or cluttered space can hamper movement.

Ergonomics for staff:
Ergonomics is about how workers interact with their work environment. Poor ergonomics can lead to injury, fatigue and other health problems.
2. Challenges :
> **Patient handling:** Lifting, moving or helping patients can be physically demanding and increase the risk of musculoskeletal injury.
> **Inadequate equipment:** Beds, chairs or other non-ergonomic equipment can cause stress or injury.
> **Awkward postures:** Nursing often involves bending, squatting or maintaining a posture for long periods.

High speed: The fast pace of work and stress can exacerbate the problems associated with poor ergonomics.

Solutions :

Training: Train staff in techniques for lifting and moving patients safely.

Adapted equipment: Invest in adjustable beds, patient lifts and other tools to facilitate mobility.

Layout: Designing workspaces that minimise the need for repetitive movements or uncomfortable postures.

Breaks and rotation: Rotate tasks and take regular breaks to avoid physical overload.

The focus on patient mobility and staff ergonomics is not just about well-being, but also about safety and efficiency. By addressing these challenges, healthcare organisations can improve the quality of care, increase patient and staff satisfaction, and reduce the costs associated with injury and absence.

Chapter 12:
MANAGEMENT SPECIFIC SITUATIONS

Poli-pathological patients.

Poli-pathological patients, also known as polymorbid or pluripathological patients, are those who suffer from a number of chronic or acute conditions at the same time. These patients require specific care, as the combination of their illnesses can lead to complications, influence therapeutic choices and make overall management more complex.

Characteristics of poly-pathological patients :
Simultaneous presence of several conditions: These conditions may be chronic, such as diabetes, hypertension or chronic obstructive pulmonary disease, or acute, such as an infection or fracture.

Drug interactions: Taking medicines for different conditions at the same time can lead to interactions, increasing the risk of adverse reactions.

Complexity of monitoring: Monitoring several conditions may require regular consultations with different specialists and coordination between them.

Challenges of care :
Global assessment: It is crucial to understand how each condition influences the others, which requires a holistic assessment.

Treatment planning: The choice of drugs and interventions must take account of all the conditions, avoiding interactions and contraindications.

Close follow-up: These patients may require more frequent follow-up to monitor the progress of their conditions and adjust treatment accordingly.

Interdisciplinary communication: Effective communication between healthcare professionals is essential to ensure coordinated care.

The role of the nurse with poly-pathological patients :

Patient education: Nurses can play a key role in educating patients about their various conditions and associated treatments.

Monitoring: Nurses must be vigilant for signs of decompensation or drug interactions.

Care coordination: The nurse can help coordinate consultations and interventions, ensuring that all carers are aware of all the patient's conditions.

Emotional support: Poli-pathological patients may feel anxious or depressed about the complexity of their situation. Nurses can offer emotional support and refer patients to appropriate resources.

The management of poly-pathological patients is a challenge in internal medicine, requiring a comprehensive and coordinated approach. Nurses play a central role in this care, offering both clinical care and emotional support to these patients.

Care for elderly patients.

The management of elderly patients in internal medicine is an essential topic, given the growing elderly population in many parts of the world. Elderly patients present unique challenges due to the complexity of their medical needs, the frequent presence of co-morbidities and the psychosocial aspects associated with ageing.

Characteristics of elderly patients :

Multiple pathology: Many elderly patients suffer from several conditions at the same time.

Physical vulnerability: With age, the body becomes more vulnerable to infection, injury and complications.

Reduced cognitive function: Some patients may show signs of dementia or other cognitive disorders.

Psychosocial aspects: isolation, depression, dependence or loss of autonomy can influence their state of health.

Challenges of care :

Overall approach: The complexity of needs requires an overall assessment, not just of obvious conditions.

Drug interactions: Taking several drugs at the same time may increase the risk of interactions and side effects.

Psychosocial considerations: Factors such as isolation or depression can affect recovery and need to be addressed.

Communication: Hearing, visual or cognitive impairments can hamper effective communication.

The role of the nurse with elderly patients :

Holistic assessment: Beyond medical needs, the nurse assesses social, emotional and functional needs.

Education and support: Explaining treatments, helping with medication management and offering support for self-care.

Falls prevention: Implementing strategies to minimise the risk of falls, a common problem among the elderly.

Liaising with families: Communicating with relatives to ensure support at home and a clear understanding of the medical situation.

Specific solutions :

Integrated geriatrics: working with geriatricians to focus on the elderly patient.

Adaptations : Use of tools such as hearing aids or reading glasses when communicating.

Medication: Regularly assess the appropriateness and safety of all medication prescribed.

Caring for elderly patients in internal medicine requires sensitivity, expertise and a holistic approach. Nurses, by being at the forefront of care, play a central role in ensuring that these patients receive appropriate, respectful and coordinated care.

Patients with special needs (disabilities, psychiatric disorders).

The care of patients with special needs, such as those with disabilities or psychiatric disorders, requires particular sensitivity and a tailored approach. These patients may require special care and attention, particularly in the context of internal medicine, where they may also have concomitant medical conditions.

Characteristics of patients with special needs :
- **Diversity of needs: The** spectrum of psychiatric disabilities and disorders is vast, ranging from physical disabilities to mood, anxiety or psychotic disorders.
- **Medical co-morbidities:** These patients may also have medical conditions that require treatment in internal medicine.
- **Communication barriers:** Patients may have difficulty communicating their needs, feelings or symptoms, whether due to a cognitive or sensory disability or a psychiatric disorder.

Challenges of care :
- **Individualised approach:** Every patient is unique and requires an approach tailored to their specific needs.

Adapted communication: It may be necessary to use alternative or adapted methods of communication, such as sign language or visual aids.

Stigma and prejudice: These patients may be confronted with stereotypes or preconceived ideas that can influence their care.

The nurse's role with patients with special needs :

Active listening: It is crucial to take the time to listen to the patient, to understand their needs and to ensure that these needs are taken into account.

Adaptation of care: This may include modifications to the environment, tools or techniques to ensure that the patient is comfortable and safe.

Liaison with specialists: Collaboration with specialists, such as psychiatrists, therapists or social workers, for comprehensive care.

Education and support: Providing clear and accessible information on treatment, and offering emotional support.

Specific solutions :

Continuing training: Nurses can benefit from specific training to better understand and meet the needs of patients with disabilities or psychiatric disorders.

Adapted equipment: Use specific equipment to facilitate care.

Communication strategies: Developing adapted communication skills, based on the patient's specific needs.

Caring for patients with special needs in internal medicine requires a patient-centred approach, characterised by humanity and respect. By listening, adapting and collaborating with other healthcare professionals, nurses can provide quality care and significantly improve the quality of life of these patients.

Chapter 13:
END-OF-LIFE MANAGEMENT
AND PALLIATIVE CARE

Communication about the end of life.

Communicating about the end of life is undoubtedly one of the most delicate and complex tasks in the medical field. It requires great sensitivity, a deep respect for the patient and his or her family, and a clear understanding of the medical, ethical and personal issues at stake.

Context and issues :
- **A crucial moment:** the end of life is a time of intense emotion, reflection and questioning for patients, their families and the care team.
- **Complex decisions:** This is often the time when important decisions need to be made about treatment, palliative care or the patient's wishes.
- **Varied emotions:** Fear, sadness, anger, resignation or even hope may be present, and each individual reacts differently.

Fundamental principles of communication :
- **Empathy:** Putting yourself in the shoes of the patient and their family, understanding their emotions and needs.
- **Honesty:** Providing clear and truthful information, while remaining sensitive.
- **Listening:** Giving patients and their families time to express themselves, ask questions and share their feelings.

Tips for effective communication :

Preparation: Before tackling the subject, it's essential to prepare yourself mentally, gather all the relevant information and choose the right time and place.

Use clear language: avoid complex medical jargon and ensure that the information is understood.

Encourage questions: Give the family and the patient the opportunity to ask questions and express their concerns.

Emotional validation: Recognising and validating the patient's and family's emotions, showing understanding and support.

Specific challenges :

Differences of opinion: Sometimes the patient, the family and the medical team may have differing opinions on the best approach.

Beliefs and values: Respect religious, cultural and personal beliefs that may influence decisions.

Managing your own emotions: As a healthcare professional, it is also crucial to recognise and manage your own emotions at the end of life.

Communication around the end of life is an art that requires delicacy, patience and deep respect. By putting the patient and family at the centre of the conversation, by listening and offering emotional support, nurses and the medical team can help navigate this difficult period with dignity and compassion.

Patient support
and his family.

Supporting patients and their families is an essential part of medical care, particularly at critical moments or when dealing with serious pathologies. This support goes beyond the simple clinical framework to encompass emotional, psychological and social aspects. It is an art that requires sensitivity, dedication and a multidisciplinary approach.

Understanding needs :
Emotional   needs: Illness or trauma can give rise to a variety of feelings, such as fear, anger, depression or acceptance. The care team must be attentive to these emotions and offer appropriate support.

Information needs: Patients and their families often want to understand the disease, treatment options, prognosis, etc. It is therefore vital to provide them with clear, honest and understandable information. It is therefore vital to provide them with clear, honest and understandable information.

Practical needs: This may include issues relating to the cost of treatment, the organisation of daily life, the care of other family members, etc.

Support strategies :
Active listening: It is crucial to give patients and their families time to express themselves, ask questions and share their feelings.

Open communication: Encouraging sincere dialogue, avoiding medical jargon and ensuring that the information shared is understood.

Psychological support: Sometimes the support of a professional such as a psychologist or psychiatrist can be beneficial.

Referral: guiding families to useful resources such as support groups, associations or social services.

Role of the care team :
Personalised care: Every patient and every family is unique. The approach must therefore be tailored to their needs and circumstances.

Training and education: The medical team must be trained in best practice in communication and support.

Interdisciplinary collaboration: The involvement of different professionals (doctors, nurses, social workers, psychologists) can offer comprehensive and diversified support.

Peer support: Team members may also need support, especially after particularly challenging situations.

Support beyond the hospital :

Discharge plan: Preparing and coordinating the patient's discharge from hospital to ensure a smooth transition to home or another institution.

Long-term follow-up: Even after discharge, regular contact points can help monitor the patient's progress and answer any emerging questions.

Bereavement support: In situations where the patient dies, offer support to the family to help them through the bereavement process.

Support for patients and their families goes beyond the simple provision of medical care. It is a holistic approach that embraces all facets of the human experience of illness, leading to a better quality of life and greater resilience in the face of health challenges.

Comfort care and pain management.

Comfort care and pain management are two of the fundamental pillars of medical care, especially in internal medicine where patients can present complex and often interconnected symptoms. The aim of this care is not only to improve patients' quality of life, but also to guarantee their dignity, regardless of the severity of their illness.

Understanding pain :
Pain can be acute, occurring suddenly in response to an injury or other cause, or chronic, often persisting for

months or even years. It can be physical in nature, but can also have emotional and psychological components.

Pain assessment :

Regular and thorough assessment is crucial. This can be done using pain scales, interviews and observations. Every patient will express and experience pain differently, hence the importance of an individualised approach.

Pain management strategies :

- **Pharmacological:** This includes the use of analgesics, anti-inflammatories, opiates and other drugs depending on the nature of the pain.
- **Non-pharmacological therapies:** such as physiotherapy, osteopathy, acupuncture, relaxation and meditation.

Comfort care :

Going beyond pain means ensuring that patients feel comfortable, respected and listened to.

- **Environment :** A clean, quiet room with the right amount of light and a pleasant temperature.
- **Basic needs:** such as ensuring proper hydration and nutrition and helping with hygiene.
- **Emotional support**: Active listening, a reassuring presence and open communication are essential.
- **Mental stimulation:** Encourage activities that stimulate the mind, such as reading, music or games.

Interdisciplinarity :

Collaboration between different professionals (doctors, nurses, psychologists, physiotherapists) is essential for comprehensive care.

Ethical challenges :

Dilemmas can sometimes arise, particularly concerning the use of opiates or decision-making at the end of life. These situations require ethical reflection and dialogue with the patient and his or her family.

Pain management and comfort care are much more than simple medical interventions. They are profoundly human endeavours which, when properly carried out, reaffirm the dignity, respect and fundamental right of every individual to a life free of unnecessary pain and as comfortable as possible. In internal medicine, where complexity is the norm, this care is all the more essential.

Chapter 14:
THE ADMINISTRATIVE ASPECT AND CASE MANAGEMENT

Documentation : why and how?

In the complex world of internal medicine, documentation plays a vital role. It serves not only as a memory, a means of communication and a source of evidence, but also as a tool for improving the quality of care. Let's take a look at why and how documentation is essential, and how it can be optimised.

Why document?

Written record: Documentation creates a written record of the patient's clinical history, progress, proposed treatments, interventions carried out and recommendations.

Communication between professionals: This ensures continuity of care by facilitating the transmission of essential information between the various healthcare professionals involved in patient care.

Decision-making support: Having a detailed medical history means that informed decisions can be made about future interventions, taking into account the patient's past progress.

Legal responsibility: Documentation serves as proof in the event of a dispute or the need to justify actions taken. It guarantees the transparency of medical actions.

Research and training: When medical records are anonymised, they can be used for clinical studies, thereby improving medical knowledge. They are also used for educational purposes to train new professionals.

How to document?

Accuracy: It is essential that information is accurate. Use appropriate medical terms, avoid ambiguity and ensure that everything is clearly explained.

Completeness: Everything relevant to the patient must be documented: symptoms, observations, test results, interventions, reactions, etc.

Organisation: Information should be presented logically and follow a recognisable structure. Use subheadings, bulleted lists and paragraphs to structure the content.

Regular updating: Records must be updated after each consultation, intervention or change in the patient's condition.

Confidentiality: Ensuring the protection of patient data. Only authorised persons should have access to documentation, and all information must be stored securely.

Use of technology: With the advent of electronic medical records, entering information is easier, more structured and more secure. Using these tools also makes it easier to find and share information.

Documentation in internal medicine, as in other medical disciplines, is a crucial task. It requires rigour, care and organisation. But its importance to the quality of care, communication between professionals and legal protection makes it a central responsibility for all those involved in healthcare.

Management electronic medical records.

The advent of electronic medical records (EMRs) has transformed the way healthcare professionals store, access and use patients' medical information. While these systems offer many benefits, they also require careful management to ensure security, efficiency and compliance.

Advantages of EMRs :

- **Quick access:** EMRs provide quick and easy access to patient information, making it easier to make informed care decisions.
- **Real-time updates:** Changes or additions to information are immediately available to all authorised healthcare professionals.
- **Reduced errors:** Electronic data entry reduces the risk of handwritten errors, making the document easier to read and reducing misunderstandings.
- **Saving resources:** EMRs can reduce the need for paper, storage space and time spent managing files.
- **Integration and communication:** EMRs can be integrated with other systems, such as laboratories or pharmacies, for seamless communication between different departments.

EMR management challenges :

- **Training:** Users must be trained in the safe and effective use of EMRs.
- **Security:** As medical information is sensitive, it is crucial to guarantee data security, both in terms of access and protection against external threats.
- **Regulatory compliance:** EMRs must comply with local and national data protection regulations.
- **Cost:** Systems can be expensive to set up, maintain and update.
- **Interfacing:** Not all EMRs are compatible with each other, which can cause problems when patients are managed by several institutions or specialists.

Good management practices :

- **Regular updates:** Keeping your system up to date is essential if you are to benefit from the latest features and security measures.

- **Controlled access:** Only authorised professionals should have access to patient information. The use of strong passwords, two-factor authentication and other security measures is recommended.
- **Backups:** Regular backups are vital to prevent data loss in the event of system failure.
- **Ongoing training:** Training should not be a one-off event. As the system is updated and standards evolve, regular training is necessary.
- **Evaluation and feedback:** Encouraging users to provide feedback on the system and its functionality can help identify areas for improvement.

Electronic medical records have revolutionised the way healthcare is delivered and managed. However, they require careful management to ensure that they are used optimally and securely. Training, awareness and open communication between EMR users and managers are essential to their success.

Legal aspects and information retention.

In the healthcare sector, the manipulation of patient data is not simply a question of efficiency or convenience. It is intimately linked to ethical and legal issues. The storage and disclosure of medical information has profound implications for privacy, patient rights and professional liability.

Legal basis :
- **Data protection laws:** These laws have been drawn up to guarantee the confidentiality and security of personal data. In the medical field, these rules are even stricter given the sensitive nature of the information.

Informed consent: Before carrying out tests, treatments or interventions, healthcare professionals must obtain the patient's informed consent. This also includes access to and storage of medical data.

Patients' rights: Patients have the right to access their medical records, to request corrections and to know who has accessed their information.

Retention of information :

Duration: National or regional laws often specify the length of time for which medical records must be kept. This period may vary depending on the nature of the information, the age of the patient or the type of treatment.

Format: With digitisation, most files are stored electronically, but their format must ensure long-term accessibility and legibility.

Security: Medical records must be kept securely to prevent unauthorised access, loss, destruction or disclosure.

Professional implications :

Liability: In the event of a breach of confidentiality or error in data processing, healthcare professionals and institutions may be held liable.

Training: Medical staff must be regularly trained and informed about the legal and ethical aspects of managing medical records.

Clear protocols: It is essential to have clear procedures and protocols for accessing, storing, disclosing and destroying medical records.

Managing medical information is not just about operational efficiency. It encompasses a profound responsibility towards patients, respect for their rights and maintaining trust in the healthcare system. Healthcare professionals must navigate this complex landscape with care, always putting the interests and rights of the patient first.

Chapter 15:
RELATIONSHIPS
WITH PATIENTS' FAMILIES

The importance of communication and education.

Communication and education are two of the cornerstones of medicine, especially when it comes to patient care. Beyond the simple exchange of information, they make a significant contribution to improving care, establishing a relationship of trust between patient and healthcare professional, and to the general well-being of the patient.

Communication is much more than an exchange of information:

Establishing trust: Transparent and open communication is essential to establish a relationship of trust between the carer and the patient. It is this trust that enables patients to feel understood and respected, and to have confidence in the medical decisions taken.

Understanding the patient: Good communication enables professionals to better understand the patient's concerns, fears and expectations, which is crucial if they are to offer appropriate care.

Therapeutic education: Through effective communication, carers can educate patients about their illness, the treatments on offer and the behaviours they should adopt to improve their state of health.

Education, an essential tool for patients :

Patient autonomy: Through education, patients acquire knowledge that enables them to better understand their illness and treatment, and thus make informed decisions about their health.

- **Prevention:** Education plays a key role in preventing illness and complications. By teaching patients about risk behaviour and preventive measures, we can reduce the incidence of certain diseases.
- **Improved adherence to treatment:** An educated patient is better able to understand the importance of following his or her treatment, which increases the effectiveness of the treatment.
- **Reducing hospital admissions**: Educating patients about warning signs and symptom management at home can reduce the number of unnecessary hospital admissions.

Medicine is not just about techniques and medicines. It is also, and above all, about people. Communication and education are essential if we are to put patients at the heart of the care we provide, making them active players in their own health and thereby improving the quality of care. It is only by truly understanding patients' needs, fears and aspirations, and by educating them appropriately, that we can move towards truly patient-centred medicine.

Managing expectations and concerns.

In the medical field, patients often arrive with a multitude of expectations and concerns. These feelings may relate to their illness, the treatments, the expected results, or even the relationship with the nursing staff. Managing these expectations and worries is not just a matter of compassion, it is also essential for the patient's well-being and the success of the treatment.

The origin of expectations and concerns :

- **Varied sources of information:** In the digital age, patients have access to a wealth of information online, from testimonials to medical articles and forums. While this abundance can be beneficial, it can also be a source of confusion and anxiety.
- **Past experiences:** Previous medical experiences, whether positive or negative, greatly influence patients' current expectations and concerns.
- **Fear of the unknown:** Not understanding an illness or treatment can lead to fear and uncertainty.

Strategies for managing expectations :

- **Active listening:** Taking the time to listen to patients, without interrupting them, helps us to better understand their expectations and adjust them if necessary.
- **Education:** Informing patients in a clear and accessible way about their disease, the treatments available, their benefits and their risks.
- **Setting realistic goals:** It is essential to clarify what the patient can expect from the treatment and what can only be hoped for.

Approaches to allaying concerns :

- **Validating emotions:** Acknowledging and validating the patient's concerns is the first step in building a relationship of trust.
- **Transparent communication:** Being honest about the risks, benefits, unknowns and alternatives helps patients to feel respected and involved in their care.
- **Psychological support:** In some cases, the support of a psychologist or social worker can be beneficial in helping patients to manage their anxiety.

Patients' expectations and concerns, if not properly addressed, can have negative consequences for medical care, ranging from non-adherence to treatment to a deterioration in mental health. On the other hand,

123

respectful, empathetic and well-informed care can transform these challenges into opportunities, strengthening the carer-patient relationship and optimising medical outcomes.

The role of the family in care and the patient's recovery.

The family plays a central role in a patient's care, particularly in internal medicine, where pathologies can be chronic, complex and affect individuals at various stages of life. Their role often goes beyond simple emotional support, encompassing day-to-day care, medical decision-making and convalescence management.

1. Emotional and psychological support :

A reassuring presence: The simple presence of a family member in hospital or during a consultation can be of immense comfort to the patient.

Listening and understanding: The family can help to de-dramatise certain situations, listen to the patient's concerns and reassure them.

2. Active participation in care :

Medication reminders: Family members can help ensure that prescriptions are followed, by reminding patients to take their medication or monitoring for any side effects.

Daily care: For patients needing assistance (washing, meals), the family can step in, sometimes offering more personalised care than in hospital.

Rehabilitation and exercise: The family can encourage and assist the patient in rehabilitation activities, which are essential for a speedy recovery.

3. Medical decision-making :

Spokesperson: If the patient is unable to communicate, the family can express their wishes and concerns to the medical team.

Joint decisions: In certain complex situations, the family, in consultation with the doctors, may have to make important decisions about treatment.

4. Convalescence management :

Post-hospitalisation care: Returning home may require adjustments (adapting the house, acquiring medical equipment). The family plays a key role in this transition.

Medical follow-up: Ensuring that appointments, follow-up examinations and post-hospitalisation instructions are respected is often made easier by family involvement.

5. Mediator between the patient and the medical team :

Clarification and questions: The family can ask questions and seek clarification, thereby facilitating mutual understanding between the patient and care staff.

Feedback: Because they are close to the patient, family members can provide valuable feedback on the patient's state of health, the effects of treatment and general well-being.

The family's presence and commitment strengthen the bond of trust between the patient and the medical team. They provide invaluable support, both emotionally and practically. Recognising and valuing their role is essential for holistic, patient-centred care. However, it is also crucial to strike a balance between the patient's needs, the family's ability to get involved and respect for the well-being of all concerned.

Chapter 16:
PATIENT SAFETY

Medical errors :
how can they be prevented?

Despite constant advances in medicine and the rigour of healthcare professionals, medical errors remain a worrying reality. While they can have dramatic consequences, it is essential to adopt a proactive approach to preventing them, rather than simply reacting after they have occurred.

1. Continuing education :
   - **Updating your knowledge:** Medicine is constantly evolving. So it's essential for healthcare professionals to continue learning throughout their careers.
   - **Training in new technologies:** Technological innovations, such as medical equipment or records management software, require appropriate training to avoid operating errors.
2. Effective communication :
   - **Between professionals:** Good communication between doctors, nurses, pharmacists and other members of the care team is crucial to avoid misunderstandings and errors.
   - **With the patient: It** is essential to understand the patient's medical history and current symptoms, and to ensure that they understand their treatment and instructions.
3. Double check :
   - **Drug prescriptions:** Before administering a drug, it is essential to check not only the drug itself, but also the dose, the route of administration and the patient's identity.

Invasive procedures: Double-checking, such as confirming the correct side of a surgery, can prevent serious errors.

4. Standardised protocols :

Clear, standardised procedures can reduce variability and therefore the risk of error. This includes checklists for certain procedures or interventions.

5. Efficient information systems :

Electronic medical records: These provide better patient follow-up, immediate availability of information and reduce the risk of errors associated with reading handwriting.

Automatic alerts: Many medical software packages can now alert professionals if an abnormal dose or drug interaction is prescribed.

6. Safety culture :

Feedback: Instead of blaming, it's more productive to analyse the mistakes that have been made and learn from them.

Incident reporting: Encouraging staff to report any errors or near-misses can help to identify weak points in the system and correct them.

7. Patient involvement :

Education: An informed patient is better able to understand his or her treatment, ask relevant questions and report any abnormalities.

Checks: Encourage patients to always check the medicines they are given or the instructions they receive.

The prevention of medical errors is based on a systemic approach, integrating both processes and individuals. While recognising the importance of individual expertise, it emphasises communication, standardisation and a culture of safety to guarantee the best possible quality of care.

The importance of protocols and checklists.

The medical world, with its complex nature and potentially life-threatening consequences, demands unfailing rigour. To guarantee the best possible care for patients and avoid medical errors, the introduction of protocols and checklists has proved to be extremely effective. But why are these tools so essential in medical practice?

1. Structuring the medical approach :
Protocols define a series of standardised steps based on the best available scientific evidence. They guide the practitioner through a succession of actions, assessments and decisions to ensure an optimal level of care.

2. Reducing human error :
Oversights, distractions and misunderstandings are inherent in human nature. Checklists act as safety nets, ensuring that every critical step is completed, thereby reducing the risk of omissions.

3. Consistent care :
Protocols ensure uniformity in patient care. Whether you are being treated by a senior doctor or a resident, in a city hospital or an academic centre, the approach should be similar if a protocol is in place.

4. Facilitating interprofessional communication :
Checklists, in particular, act as communication tools, ensuring that the whole team is synchronised and informed of the crucial stages of a procedure or care.

5. Training and education :
Protocols are excellent teaching tools for students and young professionals. They provide a clear roadmap for

understanding best practice and the underlying reasons for each step.

6. Evaluation and continuous improvement :
By documenting and following protocols, medical facilities can collect valuable data on the quality of their care. This data can then be analysed to identify areas for improvement and update protocols accordingly.

7. Strengthening patient confidence :
Patients who know that their care is based on proven protocols may have greater confidence in the healthcare system. They perceive that their care is based on a rigorous methodology rather than on ad hoc decisions.

8. Legality and liability :
In the event of complications or disputes, having followed a recognised protocol can attest to the health professional's quality approach, showing that he or she has taken all the necessary precautions to ensure patient safety.

Protocols and checklists are not simply lists or instructions to be followed. They represent a synthesis of the best current medical knowledge, combined with a recognition of the need to counter the weaknesses inherent in the human condition. Adopting these tools means adopting an approach based on excellence, focused on the well-being and safety of the patient.

Managing medicines
and preventing interactions.

In the world of medicine, drugs play an essential role in treating, curing, preventing and relieving symptoms. But their effectiveness is not without risk. Proper management of medicines and prevention of drug interactions are crucial to ensuring patient safety and optimising the effectiveness of treatment.

1. Understanding drug interactions :
A drug interaction occurs when the effect of one drug is altered by another drug, food, drink or even a medical condition.

2. Importance of pharmacological knowledge :
Knowledge of the pharmacological properties of drugs is essential to anticipate their potential effects, their metabolism, and therefore their possible interactions.

3. Polypharmacy, a growing problem :
With increasing life expectancy, many patients, particularly the elderly, are being treated for several conditions at the same time, increasing the risk of interactions.
4. Use of management tools :
Up-to-date databases and prescribing software can help identify potential drug interactions before they become a problem.

5. Communication, the cornerstone of prevention :
It is imperative that patients inform their healthcare professionals of all the medicines they are taking, including over-the-counter medicines, food supplements and herbal remedies.

6. The pivotal role of the nurse :
The nurse, as the last link before the drug is administered, plays an essential role in checking compliance with the prescription and detecting potential interactions.

7. Patient education and awareness :
It is vital to educate patients about the importance of following their prescriptions to the letter, reporting any side-effects, and consulting before adding or removing a drug.

8. Regular monitoring :
When a patient is taking several medications, regular monitoring by the doctor, with blood tests if necessary, can detect anomalies potentially linked to drug interactions.

9. Prevention rather than cure:
Prevention requires ongoing training for healthcare professionals, updating their knowledge and using available resources to anticipate interactions.

Managing medicines and preventing drug interactions are constant challenges in the world of healthcare. Collaboration between the various players in the healthcare sector, training, the use of technological tools and effective communication with patients are all key to ensuring safe and efficient medication.

Chapter 17:
HOSPITAL-ACQUIRED INFECTIONS

Prevention and management

Prevention and management in internal medicine are essential to anticipate, avoid and treat complications and health problems. They encompass a range of activities from awareness-raising to best medical practice. Here's a fluid exploration of this central notion.

The world of internal medicine is constantly evolving, with new discoveries emerging every day, new diseases being identified and existing treatments being refined. At the heart of this dynamic, two elements remain fundamental: prevention and management.

1. Prevention: the art of anticipation
Prevention is often seen as a simple hygiene or lifestyle measure. However, it goes much deeper than that. It encompasses :

  Regular check-ups: Annual check-ups can detect many conditions before they become critical.

  Vaccination: Vaccination protects against many serious diseases, not just childhood illnesses.

  Health education: Informing patients about the risks associated with certain behaviours or exposures is vital.

2. Management: responsiveness to the unexpected
Management is based on the healthcare professional's ability to react to a given situation, whether it's an acute crisis or a chronic condition.

  Medical protocols: These provide a framework for the effective treatment of a disease, based on the latest scientific data available.

Multidisciplinary care: For complex pathologies, the involvement of several specialists is often necessary.

3. Prevention and management: two sides of the same coin
They complement and reinforce each other. Good management allows effective preventive measures to be put in place. Conversely, successful prevention reduces the need for major medical interventions.

4. The challenges of the future
With the emergence of new technologies, such as telemedicine, and a better understanding of human genetics, internal medicine is on the cusp of a revolution. Prevention could be personalised according to each individual's genetic profile, and disease management could be facilitated by increasingly sophisticated digital tools.

Prevention and management are at the heart of internal medicine. They symbolise the balance between anticipation and reaction, between know-how and experience. In a world where medicine is constantly evolving, they will remain the pillars on which healthcare professionals rely to offer the best possible care to their patients.

Hygiene protocols.

At the heart of internal medicine, a discipline that encompasses the comprehensive care of adult patients suffering from a variety of often complex pathologies, the issue of hygiene is central. This concern goes beyond mere comfort: it is a real weapon against nosocomial infections, i.e. hospital-acquired infections that did not manifest themselves or were not incubating at the time of admission.

1. Hygiene issues in internal medicine

Compliance with hygiene protocols in internal medicine is crucial for several reasons:

Reducing the risk of infection: Internal medicine often treats fragile or immunocompromised patients, for whom a nosocomial infection could be extremely serious.

Patient confidence: A clean service and compliance with hygiene rules by nursing staff are guarantees of quality and professionalism.

Protection of healthcare staff : Hygiene protocols protect not only patients, but all healthcare professionals.

2. The main hygiene measures

Hand washing: This remains the cornerstone of the prevention of nosocomial infections. It must be carried out systematically before and after any contact with a patient or their environment.

Wearing personal protective equipment (PPE): Masks, gloves, gowns or safety glasses must be used depending on the situation.

Maintenance of premises: Regular cleaning with appropriate disinfectants is essential.

Waste management : Waste sorting, storage and disposal must follow strict protocols to avoid any risk of contamination.

Disinfecting medical equipment: All equipment that comes into contact with a patient must be thoroughly cleaned and sterilised if necessary.

3. The importance of training and awareness-raising

Compliance with hygiene protocols requires regular training of care staff. Frequent reminders, practical workshops and regular updating of protocols are essential to guarantee their effectiveness. It is also essential to raise awareness among patients and their families, so that they can become fully involved in the process.

Hygiene protocols in internal medicine are not simply administrative directives: they reflect a constant desire to protect the patient, guarantee the quality of care and preserve the health of the carers. At a time when antibiotic resistance is becoming a major public health issue, their importance is more crucial than ever.

Antibiotic resistance
and its impact on internal medicine.

Antibiotic resistance, a major global public health concern, is having a major impact on internal medicine. This discipline, which diagnoses and treats a multitude of often complex pathologies in adults, is facing increasing challenges from the emergence of resistant bacterial strains. To fully understand the scale of this challenge and its impact on internal medicine, an in-depth immersion is required.

1. Understanding antibiotic resistance
Over time, with the intensive and often inappropriate use of antibiotics, certain bacteria have developed defence mechanisms, rendering these drugs ineffective. This ability to adapt is natural, but it has been amplified by over-prescription, poor patient compliance and the use of antibiotics in agriculture.
2. The challenges for internal medicine
Diagnostic complexity: Faced with increasing resistance, choosing the right antibiotic requires more detailed tests to determine the bacterium's sensitivity.
Longer treatment times: To combat resistant bacteria effectively, treatments can be longer and more costly.

- **Increased risk of complications**: With less effective treatments, the risk of complications and associated morbidity increases.
- **Emergence of highly resistant strains**: Some bacteria, such as carbapenemase-producing Enterobacteriaceae (EPC), have become resistant to almost all available antibiotics.

3. Direct impact on internal medicine

By treating patients who are often fragile or even immunocompromised, internal medicine is faced with infections that are more difficult to control. Hospitalisation can be prolonged, and recourse to "last resort" antibiotics sometimes becomes the only option, with an increased risk of side-effects.

4. Solutions tailored to the context of internal medicine

- **Promote rational prescribing**: Limit the use of antibiotics to situations where they are really necessary.
- **Raising awareness and educating**: Patients and all healthcare staff need to be informed of the risks associated with overuse of antibiotics.
- **Reinforcing hygiene measures**: To prevent the spread of resistant strains, hygiene protocols must be rigorously applied.
- **Investing in research**: New antibiotics, as well as alternatives to antibiotics, need to be developed to meet this challenge.

Antibiotic resistance has a profound impact on internal medicine, putting the lives of many patients at risk and complicating the work of healthcare professionals. Faced with this challenge, a global approach combining prevention, education and innovation is essential to preserve the effectiveness of these essential medicines.

Chapter 18:
TREATMENT EMERGENCY SITUATIONS

Rapid assessment and prioritisation.

In internal medicine, as in most medical disciplines, time is often a critical factor. Whether faced with an emergency or in the day-to-day management of a large number of patients, rapid assessment and prioritisation of cases are essential to providing quality care. Here is an exploration of this fundamental approach and its importance in internal medicine.

1. The importance of a rapid assessment
In the constant stream of patients entering an internal medicine department, the ability to quickly assess an individual's state of health is vital. This assessment makes it possible to:

Identifying emergencies: Some situations require immediate intervention, otherwise the patient could be in danger.

Optimise management of time and resources: By quickly identifying the needs of each patient, it is easier to allocate available resources efficiently.

Promoting appropriate treatment: A rapid assessment provides an initial diagnostic orientation, guiding the subsequent stages of treatment.

2. Prioritisation: a delicate art
Once the initial assessment has been carried out, cases need to be prioritised. There are several reasons for this:

Ensuring patient safety: Patients with the most serious symptoms or the most unstable pathologies must be given priority.

Smoother patient care: By avoiding bottlenecks and unnecessary waiting times, prioritisation ensures better management of patient flow.

Anticipating needs: By identifying in advance patients requiring specific tests or increased monitoring, it is possible to anticipate equipment and staffing requirements.

3. Tools to help with assessment and prioritisation

Numerous tools, often integrated into hospital protocols, support carers in this process:

Emergency scores: Certain scores, based on clinical and paraclinical signs, can be used to assess the degree of urgency of a situation.

Checklists: These guide staff through the initial assessment, ensuring that no crucial elements are omitted.

Management software: More and more hospitals are equipping themselves with software to improve the management of patient flows, in real time.

4. Ongoing training: a necessity

Rapid assessment and prioritisation are skills that are honed with experience. However, ongoing training plays an essential role in keeping these skills up to date, incorporating the latest advances and becoming familiar with the most recent tools.

Rapid assessment and prioritisation are cornerstones of internal medicine. Not only do they ensure patient safety, they also help to optimise care in a context where resources, both human and material, are often limited. Mastering these skills, backed up by appropriate tools and ongoing training, is the key to high-quality medicine.

Working together
with the emergency services.

Internal medicine, a speciality at the frontiers of many disciplines, is often at the heart of the hospital system. It plays a crucial role in patient care, particularly in collaboration with the emergency services. Let's take a closer look at this collaboration, which is essential to the smooth flow of care and patient safety.

1. The interface between the emergency department and the specialty
Emergency departments are a major gateway to the hospital, where a wide range of pathologies converge, from the most benign to the most serious. When a patient needs to be admitted to hospital after being assessed in A&E, he or she is often referred to internal medicine, unless a specific speciality is required. This transition must be smooth and efficient, as it may have an impact on the patient's prognosis.
2. Essential communication
The success of this collaboration depends to a large extent on clear and effective communication. This includes:

Medical reports: Emergency departments must provide a precise summary of the situation: reason for consultation, tests carried out, treatments administered and diagnostic hypotheses.

Nurse coordination: Communication between the nurses in the two departments helps to prepare patients for admission to internal medicine, anticipate their needs and ensure uninterrupted care.

Sharing information on available resources: This includes available beds, on-call staff, specific equipment, etc.

3. Training and updating skills

Emergency departments and internal medicine departments have their own specific characteristics, but cross-training can be beneficial:

Rotating internships: Enabling doctors and nurses to spend time in the other department to better understand its challenges and constraints.

Joint training: Organising training sessions on frequently encountered diseases, treatment protocols and communication tools.

4. Flow management and relieving congestion in emergency departments

Collaboration between these two services is also essential to manage the influx of patients and avoid overcrowding:

Rapid referral: Patients stabilised in emergency but requiring prolonged hospitalisation should be transferred rapidly to internal medicine.

Short-term units: These units, often run jointly by the two departments, are used to admit patients requiring additional monitoring or investigations before a decision is made to admit them to hospital or return them home.

Collaboration between internal medicine and emergency services is a cornerstone of hospital care. It ensures a safe and efficient transition for patients, while optimising the use of hospital resources. However, this collaboration is not self-evident, and requires constant efforts in terms of communication, training and coordination.

Rapid intervention protocols.

In internal medicine, as in many hospital departments, time is often of the essence. Some patients may experience a rapid deterioration in their condition, requiring immediate intervention. Rapid Response Protocols (RRPs) have been designed to meet this need, providing clear, structured guidelines for managing these urgent situations. Let's take a look at how they work and why they are essential.

1. Definition and principles of RIPs

Rapid response protocols are pre-established procedures for responding to specific situations where immediate action is required. The aim of these protocols is to standardise responses, reduce errors and improve the effectiveness of interventions.

2. Early identification of patients at risk

The key to a successful RIP is to act before the situation becomes critical. This requires :

Continuous monitoring: Vital signs and other indicators should be monitored regularly to detect any abnormalities.

Staff training: All staff, from doctors to care assistants, must be trained to recognise the warning signs of deterioration and know when to trigger a PIR.

3. Composition of the intervention team

The rapid response team is generally made up of :

A senior doctor: Usually a specialist in emergency medicine or intensive care.

A senior nurse: Experienced in dealing with emergencies.

Other professionals as required: For example, a respiratory specialist if the patient has breathing difficulties.

4. Key stages in the intervention

Initial assessment: Once on site, the team rapidly assesses the patient's condition to confirm the need for intervention.

Stabilisation: The team takes the necessary steps to stabilise the patient, whether this involves administering oxygen, medication or other interventions.

Transfer if necessary: If the patient requires more specialised care, they may be transferred to another department, such as intensive care.

5. Feedback and continuous improvement

After each operation, it is crucial to :

Analyse the intervention: Understand what worked well and identify areas for improvement.

Update the PIR if necessary: Protocols must be kept up to date and adapted in line with feedback.

Rapid response protocols are an essential element of patient safety in internal medicine. They ensure a rapid, structured and effective response to potentially critical situations, reducing risks to the patient and improving care outcomes.

Chapter 19:
NURSES AND RESEARCH

The importance of research in nursing care.

Nursing research is a cornerstone in the evolution of nursing practice, playing a vital role in ensuring quality, evidence-based care. More than simply a complement to traditional medicine, this research embodies the nursing profession's aspiration to continually improve and refine the care provided to patients.

At the heart of nursing research is a deep desire to understand not only the illnesses themselves, but also the human experience of illness. It looks at questions such as: How do patients live with their illness on a day-to-day basis? How can they be better supported emotionally, psychologically and socially? Or how can specific nursing interventions improve patient outcomes?

The impact of this research is tangible. Thanks to it, care protocols are being reviewed and adapted, offering innovative approaches that are better aligned with patients' needs. It also sheds light on the effectiveness of new interventions, enabling nurses to ensure that their practices are not only safe, but also optimal for their patients.

Nursing research also contributes to nurses' professional autonomy. By conducting and drawing on their own research, nurses do not simply follow medical guidelines, but become active players in the development of healthcare. They are able to make significant contributions to debates on best practice, reinforcing the vital role they play within medical teams.

This research also has an impact on the education and training of nurses. By incorporating the latest discoveries into study programmes, future generations of nurses are better prepared to face the challenges of an ever-changing medical landscape.

Finally, nursing research enriches our overall understanding of healthcare. It reminds us that, science and technology aside, medical care is fundamentally about people helping people. And for that, every gesture, every word, every intervention counts.

Nursing research is much more than an academic pursuit. It reflects the passion, dedication and commitment of nurses to provide the best possible evidence-based care to all those entrusted to their care.

Participation in clinical trials.

Participation in clinical trials is an essential part of today's medical landscape. The aim of these studies is to assess the efficacy and safety of new interventions, whether drugs, medical devices, therapies or surgical techniques. Nurses play a key role in these studies, and are essential to their success.

First of all, it is often the nurse who is in the front line in identifying patients eligible for a clinical study. Thanks to their close relationship with patients and their in-depth knowledge of their medical history and current state of health, nurses can effectively guide patients towards the studies that are best suited to them.

The nurse then administers the experimental treatments. This stage requires great precision and strict adherence to protocols, as any variation could affect the results of the study. The nurse must be rigorous, ensuring that each patient receives the exact treatment planned, at the right dose and at the right time.

As well as administering treatment, nurses also play a crucial role in monitoring patients. They are often the first to identify and report any side effects or complications, enabling rapid intervention to ensure patient safety. They also monitor patients on a regular basis, gathering essential data to assess the effectiveness of the treatment.

Communication is also a central component of nurses' participation in clinical trials. They are the liaison point between patients and the research team, ensuring that patients are well informed and comfortable throughout the study. They answer questions, allay concerns and ensure that patients fully understand their rights, including the right to withdraw from the study at any time.

In addition, ongoing training is essential for nurses involved in clinical studies. The medical landscape is changing rapidly, and nurses need to be up to date with the latest advances, study protocols and ethical regulations.

The participation of nurses in clinical trials is essential to advance medicine and improve patient care. Their expertise, dedication and ability to connect with patients ensure that these studies are conducted with the highest level of integrity, efficiency and care.

Contribution to progress knowledge of internal medicine.

Internal medicine is a vast and constantly evolving field, covering a multitude of pathologies and disorders. It's a field in which new discoveries are made every day, calling certainties into question, and where innovation is constant. Nurses play a major role in this dynamic, actively contributing to the development and refinement of knowledge in internal medicine.

Because of their daily proximity to patients, nurses are privileged observers of symptoms, therapeutic effects and reactions to treatments. These observations, although often informal, can reveal trends, unexpected side-effects or rare reactions to a treatment. This wealth of information, when shared and analysed, can influence clinical research and care protocols.

In addition, nurses are often involved in implementing new techniques or therapies. Their feedback on the practicality, effectiveness and obstacles encountered is invaluable in refining these methods and making them more appropriate and efficient.

Nurses are also involved in research. Many nurses are pursuing advanced training and doctorates, and are participating in or initiating clinical studies. They ask essential questions, based on their experience in the field, which can lead to new avenues of research or challenge established practices.

Interprofessional collaboration is also a vector for the advancement of knowledge. By working closely with internists, pharmacists, physiotherapists and other health professionals, nurses participate in fruitful multidisciplinary exchanges. These synergies enable a holistic approach to medical problems, promoting more integrative and personalised medicine.

Continuing education courses, conferences and symposia are all opportunities for nurses to keep abreast of the latest advances, but also to share their expertise. Their voices, their testimonies and their questions enrich the medical debate and stimulate collective reflection.

Internal medicine nurses are far more than just executors; they are key players in the advancement of knowledge. Their expertise, curiosity and commitment make them essential vectors of progress, guaranteeing ever more precise, humane medicine tailored to patients' needs.

Chapter 20:
TECHNOLOGY AND INNOVATION
IN NURSING CARE

New technologies
at the service of the patient.

In a world of constant technological change, medicine is no exception. Technological advances have revolutionised the way we approach healthcare, transforming the patient-carer relationship and opening up previously unimaginable therapeutic possibilities. In internal medicine, a rich and complex field par excellence, these innovations are particularly striking.

The era of the connected patient
Connected devices have taken over our daily lives, and the medical sector is no exception. Watches, bracelets, mobile applications, etc. enable patients to monitor parameters such as blood pressure, heart rate, blood sugar levels and physical activity in real time. When shared with healthcare professionals, this data can provide a more complete and continuous picture of the patient's condition, encouraging more personalised care.

Telemedicine: remote treatment
Telemedicine, which enables patients to be consulted remotely via videoconferencing, represents a genuine revolution, particularly for patients who are geographically isolated or have reduced mobility. It offers continuity of care, while reducing costs and travel. This technology also encourages collaboration between healthcare professionals, enabling exchanges and second opinions in real time.

Artificial intelligence and predictive medicine
AI is set to transform medicine. It offers the possibility of analysing immense quantities of data in record time, enabling the detection of trends, anomalies or patterns that the human eye would be unable to perceive. This is particularly useful in internal medicine for anticipating decompensation in chronic patients, or for personalising treatments according to an individual's genetic and biological profile.

Innovative medical devices
Connected insulin pumps, monitoring implants, intelligent respiratory assistance devices... the scope of medical devices is widening and their precision is being refined thanks to technology. These innovations enable better regulation of pathologies and improved quality of life for patients.

Ethical and security challenges
While these technologies open up promising new therapeutic horizons, they also raise ethical issues, particularly when it comes to data confidentiality. Securing this data is essential to guarantee patient confidence and prevent any risk of piracy.

Because of its complexity and richness, internal medicine benefits greatly from technological advances. These patient-centred innovations have the potential to transform our approach to healthcare, making it more precise, more humane and, above all, more effective. However, it is essential to bear in mind that technology must remain at the service of people, and not the other way round.

Telemedicine and remote monitoring.

With the rise of digital technologies, medicine has entered a phase of radical transformation. Telemedicine, in particular, has emerged as an effective solution to today's medical challenges, especially in internal medicine, where regular, in-depth patient follow-up is vital.

A world without medical borders
In the past, medical consultations were confined to the cramped confines of a doctor's surgery. Today, thanks to telemedicine, the walls are coming down. Patients in rural areas, those with reduced mobility or even those abroad can now access specialist care without having to travel.

The ultimate monitoring tool
Internal medicine often deals with chronic pathologies requiring regular monitoring. Telemedicine facilitates this monitoring by offering the possibility of regular remote consultations, enabling continuous monitoring, rapid adaptation of treatments and early detection of complications.

Interconnecting professionals
Telemedicine also encourages better communication between healthcare professionals. For example, a general practitioner can seek the advice of a specialist in real time, optimising patient care.

Safety first and foremost
While telemedicine offers many advantages, it is nonetheless subject to security concerns. The transmission of medical data must meet strict security and confidentiality standards. The platforms used for telemedicine are therefore subject to regular checks to ensure that patient information is protected.

The limits of technology
Although revolutionary, telemedicine cannot totally replace physical contact. Some examinations require face-to-face presence, and palpation, for example, remains irreplaceable. What's more, some people, particularly the elderly, may feel unsettled by this approach.

Telemedicine and remote monitoring embody the medicine of tomorrow. They make up for some of the shortcomings of the current system, offering accessibility and regular monitoring, while preserving the human relationship between patient and doctor. In internal medicine, this modern approach is proving particularly relevant, paving the way for ever more precise and individualised care.

Digital applications and tools for nurses.

The digital world has profoundly transformed the healthcare landscape. For nurses, who are often on the front line of care, these tools represent an opportunity to improve their day-to-day work, become more efficient and offer better quality care. Here's a look at how digital applications and tools are redefining the nursing profession.

Patient management and follow-up
Dedicated applications now enable nurses to monitor their patients' medical records in real time. These tools centralise information, facilitate access to essential data and help with care planning. Some software also offers the possibility of sending reminders for medication or appointments, improving patient compliance with their treatment.

Ongoing training and access to information
Continuing education is essential in the healthcare sector. Thanks to online platforms and specialised applications, nurses can now take courses, take part in webinars or consult professional resources, all at their own pace and according to their availability.

Reinforced communication
Communication is a cornerstone of nursing care. Digital tools such as secure messaging and telemedicine platforms enable fluid communication between different healthcare professionals, as well as with patients. This

means better coordination of care and more holistic treatment.

Assistance with care

A host of applications are now helping nurses to carry out their day-to-day tasks. From dosage calculators and procedure guides to manuals on the use of specific equipment, these digital tools are becoming invaluable allies in clinical practice.

Well-being and stress management

Nursing can be a stressful profession. Fortunately, a number of applications focusing on meditation, time management or even psychological support are available to help healthcare professionals manage the emotional and mental challenges of their profession.

Digital applications and tools for nurses are not just technological gadgets; they are genuine extensions of nurses' skills and knowledge. Used properly, they can transform patient care, improve the quality of care and reinforce the central role of nurses in the healthcare pathway. However, it is crucial to be trained in their use and to remain critical of their relevance to ensure that they are used ethically and safely.

Chapter 21:
COMPLEMENTARY APPROACHES IN INTERNAL MEDICINE

Complementary integrated therapies (CIT).

In internal medicine, the clinical approach is often centred on the diagnosis and treatment of underlying conditions. Increasingly, however, Western medicine is opening up to non-conventional forms of care, known as complementary integrated therapies (CIT). The aim of these therapies is to improve the patient's overall well-being, manage symptoms and optimise quality of life.

What are integrated complementary therapies?

CBT encompasses a wide range of practices, often derived from ancient medical traditions, which are used in conjunction with conventional medicine. Among the most popular are :

Acupuncture: Originating in China, acupuncture involves inserting fine needles into specific points on the body to balance vital energy and relieve pain or other symptoms.

Meditation and mindfulness: These practices help to reduce stress and anxiety and can contribute to better pain management.

Chiropractic: Centred on manual manipulation of the spinal column, it aims to improve musculoskeletal function.

Aromatherapy: uses essential oils to promote relaxation and well-being and manage certain symptoms.

Massage therapy: Therapeutic massage can help relax muscles, stimulate circulation and promote a general sense of well-being.

Integrating ICT into internal medicine

The use of ICT is not intended to replace conventional treatments, but rather to complement them. When integrated appropriately :

They can offer symptomatic relief: for example, acupuncture can reduce the nausea associated with certain treatments or chronic pain.

They promote a patient-centred approach: CBTs often encourage self-management and offer patients tools to actively participate in their own healing.

They can reduce dependence on medication: For example, meditation and massage therapy can reduce the need for painkillers in some patients.

Complementary integrated therapies offer an additional dimension to treatment in internal medicine. They recognise the importance of addressing health and well-being in a holistic way, taking into account the complex interaction between body, mind and environment. However, their integration must be carried out with discernment, always ensuring that the ICTs chosen are appropriate and safe for the patient.

Nursing care based on evidence.

In the vast world of medicine, practices are evolving at a breathtaking pace. To guarantee patient safety and provide the best possible care, it is essential that healthcare professionals rely on tried and tested methods. This is where evidence-based nursing comes in.

What is evidence-based care?

Evidence-based nursing (EBN) refers to the judicious and explicit integration of the best clinical evidence from research, combined with the clinical expertise of the nurse and the values and preferences of the patient.

The pillars of SIBP

Clinical research: This is the fundamental element of SIBP. Clinical studies, systematic reviews, meta-analyses and randomised controlled trials provide valuable information on the effectiveness of interventions.

Clinical expertise: Even in the face of the best research, the nurse's clinical experience remains essential for interpreting and applying these data in the specific context of a patient.

Patient preferences: Patient-centred care recognises that in many situations there is no single 'right' answer, and that the patient's preferences, values and needs should guide the care plan.

The importance of SIBP

Improved quality of care: SIBP ensures that patients receive care based on the most up-to-date and relevant information.

Reducing unnecessary variation in practice: Based on evidence, we can standardise care for similar situations, while adapting to individual needs.

Promoting a culture of continuous learning: SIBP encourages an attitude of perpetual learning, where nurses are always on the lookout for best practice.

Implementing SIBP
Adopting evidence-based care requires institutional and individual commitment. This includes:

Training: Nurses must be trained in research and the critical evaluation of studies.

Access to resources: The availability of databases, journals and evaluation tools is crucial.

A culture of questioning: Encouraging nurses to ask questions, to challenge established practices and to actively seek improvements.

In an ever-changing medical landscape, evidence-based nursing is a beacon, guiding professionals towards the highest possible quality of care. It combines the art of the nurse, her clinical experience, with the rigour of science, to provide optimal care for every patient.

The integration of alternative practices (acupuncture, massage, aromatherapy).

Internal medicine, which is fundamentally based on tried and tested scientific methods, is nevertheless constantly evolving, always seeking the best for the patient. In this journey towards optimal care, the integration of alternative practices, also known as complementary medicine, is becoming increasingly important. These often ancestral methods offer a holistic vision of the patient, taking into account both body and mind.

What do we mean by "alternative practices"?
Alternative or complementary medicine refers to a series of techniques and therapeutic approaches that are not an integral part of conventional medicine. These include acupuncture, therapeutic massage, aromatherapy, reflexology and meditation.

Potential benefits for internal medicine patients
Pain reduction: Techniques such as acupuncture or massage can help relieve certain types of pain, without the need for systematic use of analgesics.
Stress and anxiety management: Meditation, aromatherapy and yoga can be excellent tools for

helping patients manage the stress associated with illness or a stay in hospital.

Improving general well-being: By considering the patient as a whole, these approaches can contribute to a general feeling of well-being and harmony.

Integration into the hospital environment

Integrating these methods into the context of internal medicine requires a considered approach:

Training and awareness: It is vital that staff are trained and made aware of these practices so that they can recommend them in complete safety.

Working with experts: The involvement of specialists (certified acupuncturists, therapeutic masseurs, etc.) guarantees safe and effective treatment.

Personalised care: Every patient is unique. His or her openness to and needs for alternative therapies will vary, requiring a tailored approach.

Precautions and considerations

While these practices offer undeniable advantages, it is essential to bear in mind :

Communication: It is crucial to discuss with the patient the different options available, the expected benefits, but also the limitations of these approaches.

Avoiding interactions: Certain essential oils used in aromatherapy, for example, can interact with medicinal treatments. A rigorous assessment is therefore necessary.

Do not substitute: These practices complement conventional medicine, not replace it. Evidence-based medicine remains the mainstay of treatment.

In a medical world that is increasingly open to interdisciplinarity, the integration of alternative practices in internal medicine symbolises this desire to offer comprehensive care that respects the individuality of each patient. By combining science and tradition, modernity and ancestry, internal medicine is paving the way for increasingly holistic care.

Chapter 22:
PHARMACOLOGY
IN INTERNAL MEDICINE

Commonly used medicines.

Internal medicine, as an all-encompassing medical speciality, is concerned with the prevention, diagnosis and non-surgical treatment of various diseases in adults. As a result, a wide range of medicines are commonly used to manage a multitude of conditions. While an exhaustive list would be daunting, it is possible to highlight some common medicines, classified by category, that are often encountered in internal medicine.

1. Cardiovascular drugs

Antihypertensives: To regulate blood pressure. Examples: ACE inhibitors such as ramipril, beta-blockers such as propranolol.

Anticoagulants: To prevent the formation of blood clots. Examples: warfarin, direct oral anticoagulants such as rivaroxaban.

Anti-arrhythmics: To regulate heart rhythm. Example: amiodarone.

2. Endocrinological drugs

Antidiabetics: To manage diabetes. Examples: metformin, DPP-4 inhibitors such as sitagliptin.

Thyroid patients: Like levothyroxine for hypothyroid patients.

3. Medicines for gastrointestinal diseases

Antacids: To treat gastro-oesophageal reflux and ulcers. Example: omeprazole.

Antidiarrhoeals: such as loperamide.

4. Medicines for lung diseases
    Bronchodilators: For asthmatics and COPD patients. Examples: salbutamol, tiotropium.
    Anti-inflammatories: such as inhaled corticosteroids, budesonide.
5. Drugs for kidney disease
    Diuretics: Like furosemide, which helps to eliminate excess fluid from the body.
6. Medicines for neurological conditions
    Anticonvulsants : For epilepsy. Example: carbamazepine.
    Anti-parkinsonian drugs: Like levodopa.
7. Anti-infectives
    Antibiotics: such as amoxicillin or ciprofloxacin.
    Antivirals: Like oseltamivir for flu.
8. Pain medication
    Analgesics: such as paracetamol, ibuprofen or opioids like morphine.
9. Medicines for rheumatological conditions
    Non-steroidal anti-inflammatory drugs (NSAIDs): To treat inflammation and pain. Example: diclofenac.

Internal medicine is characterised by the wide range of diseases it treats, and this is reflected in the diversity of medicines commonly used. It is essential for nurses and internists to be familiar with these medicines, their indications, dosages, potential interactions and side effects, in order to ensure the best possible patient care.

Management drug interactions.

In internal medicine, patients often present with multiple pathologies requiring polypharmacological treatment, which increases the risk of drug interactions. A drug interaction occurs when the effect of one drug is modified by the presence of another drug, food, drink or environmental condition. These interactions can potentially be beneficial, harmful or neutralise the effect of the drug.

1. Recognition of potential interactions
- **Common sources of interactions:** Some drugs are more likely to cause interactions than others. Examples include anticoagulants, antihypertensives, antiepileptics and some antidepressants.
- **Tools and resources:** The use of electronic drug databases or specific applications can help to quickly identify potential interactions.

2. Clinical assessment of interactions
- **Severity: Not** all drug interactions are clinically significant. It is crucial to assess whether the interaction will cause harm to the patient.
- **Benefit vs. Risk:** In some cases, despite a known interaction, the benefit of the combination of drugs may outweigh the risks, provided it is closely monitored.

3. Management strategies
- **Adjusting doses:** If two drugs interact, it may be possible to adjust the dose of one or both drugs to avoid undesirable effects.
- **Changing the time of administration:** Administering drugs at different times of the day can sometimes minimise their interaction.
- **Increased monitoring:** Some drugs require regular monitoring of clinical parameters or laboratory tests to monitor the effects of the interaction.
- **Patient education:** Informing patients of the potential signs and symptoms of a drug interaction can lead to early detection.
- **Interprofessional communication:** Fluid communication between doctors, nurses, pharmacists and other healthcare professionals is

essential to effectively manage and prevent drug interactions.

4. Preventing interactions

Regular review of medicines: It is vital to review the patient's medication list regularly, particularly when a drug is added or withdrawn.

Pharmaceutical consultation: Pharmacists are trained to detect and manage drug interactions. Their expertise can be invaluable.

Managing drug interactions is a vital aspect of care in internal medicine. Due to the complexity of patients and their treatments, a proactive, educational and collaborative approach is essential to ensure safe and effective care.

Pharmacogenetics and personalised medicine.

The advent of personalised medicine has radically transformed the way internal medicine patients are treated. At the heart of this revolution is pharmacogenetics, a discipline that studies how a person's genetic variations influence their response to drugs.

1. What is pharmacogenetics?

Definition: Pharmacogenetics focuses on how individual genetic variations affect the response to drugs, enabling more targeted and precise therapy.

Genes and medicines: Many genes can influence the way a person assimilates, uses or reacts to a specific drug.

2. Why is it revolutionary?

Individualised treatment: Thanks to pharmacogenetics, drugs can be tailored specifically to a person's genetics, offering a more precise therapeutic approach that is less likely to cause adverse effects.

- **Reducing side effects:** By understanding how a person metabolises a drug, it is possible to reduce the risk of serious side effects.
- **Dose optimisation:** Pharmacogenetics can help determine the optimal dose for an individual, ensuring efficacy while reducing the risk of overdose.

3. Applications in internal medicine

- **Cardiovascular diseases:** Adapting anticoagulants and statins to genetic factors to minimise risks and maximise benefits.
- **Psychiatric disorders:** Selection of antidepressants or antipsychotics based on genetic profile to improve results and reduce side effects.
- **Pain:** Personalised pain management, particularly with opioids, to avoid over- or under-medication.
- **Autoimmune and inflammatory diseases:** Optimisation of immunosuppressants and biologics according to the expected response based on the genetic profile.

4. Challenges and ethical considerations

- **Access:** Genetic tests can be expensive and are not always reimbursed by insurance.
- **Privacy:** The protection of genetic information and the guarantee that it will not be used in a discriminatory manner are crucial.
- **Understanding:** Ensuring adequate education for patients and healthcare professionals on pharmacogenetics is essential for effective use.

5. The future of pharmacogenetics in internal medicine

- **Ongoing research:** As more and more genetic variations are discovered, the application of pharmacogenetics will continue to expand.
- **Technological integration:** Combining advanced electronic medical records with pharmacogenetic

databases can facilitate large-scale personalised medicine.

Pharmacogenetics embodies the future of internal medicine, offering care tailored to the genetic individuality of each patient. While challenges remain, the potential benefits for patient health are immense, leading to more effective and safer treatments.

Chapter 23:
THE NURSE
DEALING WITH ETHICAL SITUATIONS

Cases of conscience.

In medicine, particularly internal medicine, healthcare professionals are regularly faced with ethical dilemmas that challenge their conscience. These situations, known as cases of conscience, go to the very heart of personal, professional and societal values.

1. Nature of cases of conscience
Cases of conscience arise when medical choices conflict with ethical, moral or legal principles. For example, deciding whether to continue or stop treatment for a terminally ill patient, or choosing between two patients for the allocation of an organ for transplantation.

2. Some examples of dilemmas
   Therapeutic overkill: How far should we go in treating a seriously ill patient? When is an intervention more harmful than beneficial?
   Informed consent: How can genuine consent be obtained when the patient is unable to understand his or her medical situation?
   Confidentiality: What should be done when an adult patient asks not to inform his or her family of a serious diagnosis, such as cancer?
   Refusal of treatment: How should we react when patients refuse life-saving or life-prolonging treatment, particularly because of their religious beliefs?

3. The importance of dialogue
When faced with these dilemmas, dialogue is essential. This involves discussion with the patient and his family, as well as within the medical team. This exchange helps us to better understand the issues at stake and everyone's perspectives, and to try to find a consensus or, at the very least, a way forward that is acceptable to all the parties involved.

4. Ethics committees
Many hospitals have set up ethics committees. These committees are made up of healthcare professionals, lawyers, philosophers and sometimes patient representatives. Their role is to provide advice and recommendations on cases of conscience and ethical dilemmas submitted by healthcare professionals.

5. Training in medical ethics
To prepare healthcare professionals for these dilemmas, training in medical ethics is increasingly being incorporated into medical curricula. The aim is to give doctors and nurses the tools they need to think and act ethically when faced with the challenges of their practice.

Cases of conscience are inherent to medical practice. While each situation is unique, they all call into question the profound values of the carer, the patient and society as a whole. Faced with these dilemmas, listening, dialogue and ethical reflection are essential if we are to make informed decisions that respect human dignity.

Ethical decision-making.

Decision-making in medicine is a complex process, requiring not only scientific and clinical knowledge, but also ethical reflection. In internal medicine, where patients often present complex, multi-systemic problems, ethical decision-making is of paramount importance.

1. What is ethical decision-making?
Ethical decision-making is about reflecting on the moral values that guide our actions and decisions. It comes into play when several choices are possible and each of these choices has different ethical implications.

2. The four principles of medical ethics
Ethical decision-making in medicine is often based on four fundamental principles:

Beneficence: acting in the patient's best interests.

Non-maleficence: not harming or avoiding harm to the patient.

Autonomy: respecting patients' right to make their own decisions about their health.

Justice: treating patients fairly and distributively.

3. The challenges of ethical decision-making in internal medicine

Clinical complexity: Internal medicine patients often have complex medical problems, making decision-making more difficult and requiring a global approach.

Diversity of values: Patients, families and carers may have different beliefs, values and expectations, which can lead to ethical dilemmas.

Resource limitations: In a context of limited resources, how can we ensure equitable distribution of care?

4. Ethical deliberation
When faced with an ethical dilemma, deliberation is essential. This involves :

Gathering information: understanding the patient's medical, social and personal context.

Reflection: weigh up the benefits and risks of each option, taking ethical principles into account.
Dialogue: talking with the patient, family and healthcare team to share perspectives, understand the issues and try to reach a consensus.

5. Ethics committees
When faced with complex ethical dilemmas, ethics committees can offer valuable expertise. These multidisciplinary committees provide advice, recommendations and sometimes mediation to help healthcare teams navigate the murky waters of ethical dilemmas.

Ethical decision-making is at the heart of internal medicine. It requires careful thought, an understanding of the patient as a whole, and the ability to navigate between ethical principles, patient needs and clinical and organisational realities. The ultimate goal is always to ensure the patient's well-being, while respecting their rights and dignity.

Hospital ethics committees.

Navigating the complexities of medical decision-making often requires more than just medical knowledge. This is where hospital ethics committees come in. They act as beacons, lighting the way through sometimes murky waters, offering ethical guidance where medical choices meet moral dilemmas.

1. What is a hospital ethics committee?
A hospital ethics committee is a multidisciplinary group of healthcare professionals, philosophers, lawyers and sometimes even members of the public, who meet to discuss and advise on complex ethical issues relating to patient care.

2. The role of ethics committees

Ethical consultation: Providing recommendations on specific cases submitted by healthcare staff or management.

Education: Organise training for staff on ethical principles and their practical application.

Policy: Participate in the drafting of guidelines and protocols on ethical issues.

Research: Ensuring ethical oversight of clinical research projects carried out at the hospital.

3. The value of collective deliberation

Ethics committees draw their strength from their collective nature. By bringing together people from different disciplines, they offer a plurality of perspectives, enabling in-depth analysis of ethical situations.

4. Common dilemmas

End of life: decisions concerning the withdrawal or continuation of treatment.

Consent: situations where the patient cannot give consent.

Limited resources: allocation of resources in situations of scarcity.

Conflicts between patients and the care team: disagreements over treatment plans.

5. The challenges facing ethics committees

Diversity of opinion: managing and respecting different perspectives.

Temporality: making decisions in emergency situations.

Limits to their role: committees advise, but do not make clinical decisions.

6. The scope of ethics committees
Although their role is advisory, their impact is far-reaching. Ethics committees help to strengthen the ethical culture within hospitals, providing a forum for dialogue and reflection on sometimes sensitive issues.

In the complex world of modern medicine, where technology, humanity and ethics constantly intersect, hospital ethics committees play an essential role. They ensure that, even in the most difficult situations, the moral compass remains pointed towards the patient's best interests, while respecting ethical principles and human dignity.

Chapter 24:
RISK MANAGEMENT
IN INTERNAL MEDICINE

Identify and prevent risk situations.

In the context of internal medicine, every nurse is faced with a constant stream of diverse situations. Some are routine, others urgent, but all require constant vigilance to identify and prevent risk situations. These critical moments can have an impact on the health or even the life of the patient, but with the right training and awareness, they can be anticipated and avoided.

1. Recognising warning signs
Any experienced nurse will tell you that the ability to recognise even a subtle change in a patient is essential. Whether it's a change in heart rate, a change in skin colour or an alteration in consciousness, these clues can be the first signs of impending deterioration.

2. The importance of listening
Active listening to patients is crucial. Sometimes patients may express discomfort or a symptom which, although it may seem minor, is in fact the first sign of a complication.

3. Assessment tools
Regular use of standardised assessment tools, such as pain scales or neurological assessment scores, can help to objectivise and monitor the patient's condition, enabling early detection of risk situations.

4. Work closely with the team
Sharing information between nurses, doctors and other members of the healthcare team is vital. Information that

seems insignificant in one context may prove crucial in another. Team meetings and communications are the ideal time to share these observations.

5. Further training

Medicine is constantly evolving. Nurses need to keep abreast of the latest recommendations, techniques and protocols to anticipate the risks associated with new treatments or emerging diseases.

6. Simulations and practical exercises

Simulations of high-risk scenarios, such as haemorrhage or cardiac arrest, can help prepare the team to act quickly and effectively in real-life situations.

7. The importance of the environment

A well-organised, clean and safe environment can significantly reduce the risk of medical errors. This includes proper management of medicines, clear signposting of risk areas and the provision of protective equipment.

8. The proactive approach

Instead of waiting for a problem to occur, adopting a proactive approach means that many risk situations can be anticipated and prevented. This includes regular checks on equipment, ongoing assessment of high-risk patients, and the implementation of preventive protocols.

Preventing risk situations in internal medicine is a subtle blend of science, instinct and experience. It's a constant challenge, but with the right training, close collaboration with the care team, and constant vigilance, nurses play a decisive role in patient safety and well-being.

Reporting protocols.

In hospital settings, reporting adverse events, medical errors or potentially dangerous situations is crucial to ensuring patient safety and quality of care. In internal medicine, where patients may present with complex pathologies and multiple co-morbidities, the implementation of effective reporting protocols is all the more essential.

1. Objectives of the reporting protocols
The primary objective of reporting protocols is not to punish but to identify, understand and prevent similar situations from occurring in the future. They enable :
    Improve the quality of care.
    Identify areas at risk.
    Promote a culture of safety and transparency.

2. Types of reportable events
A variety of events can be reported:
    Medication errors (wrong dose, wrong drug).
    Post-intervention complications.
    Diagnostic errors.
    Problems with medical equipment.
    Patient safety incidents (falls, escapes).
    Any other unusual or worrying event.

3. Reporting procedures
The reporting process must be clear and accessible to all healthcare professionals:
    Use of standardised forms.
    Possibility of anonymous reporting to encourage reporting without fear of repercussions.
    Computerised systems to facilitate data collection and analysis.

4. Processing alerts

Once a report has been made, a clear procedure must be put in place for dealing with it:

- Analysis of the event by a dedicated team (usually comprising doctors, nurses, pharmacists, etc.).
- Assessment of the seriousness of the incident and its impact.
- Proposed corrective or preventive measures.
- Follow-up of recommendations and evaluation of their effectiveness.

5. Communication

Communication about reported events is essential:

- Informing patients and their families, in a fully transparent manner, when an incident affecting their care occurs.
- Organise feedback sessions within the healthcare team to share the lessons learned from incidents.

6. Training and awareness-raising

Regular training sessions on the importance of reporting and how to do it are essential to ensure the effectiveness of the system.

7. Assessment and updating

It is vital to regularly assess the effectiveness of the reporting protocols in place and to adapt them to the needs identified.

Reporting protocols are an essential tool for ensuring patient safety in internal medicine. Not only do they enable errors to be identified and remedied, they also help to create a safety culture in which every professional feels involved and responsible.

Morbidity and mortality reviews.

In the medical world, morbidity and mortality reviews (MMRs) are clinical meetings designed to analyse, in a collegial manner, the cases of patients who have suffered complications or died, with the aim of learning lessons and improving the quality of care. These reviews are essential to the continuous improvement of patient care.

1. RMM objectives

The main aim of MMRs is to turn medical errors, complications or deaths into learning opportunities for the entire healthcare team. More specifically, they enable :

Identify the causes of complications or death.

Assessing the quality of medical care.

Identify the factors contributing to adverse events.

Propose and implement improvement actions.

2. Conduct of a MMR

The RMM process is generally structured as follows:

Pre-selection of cases: The cases to be discussed are generally chosen because of their seriousness, their unusual nature or because they present a learning opportunity.

Presentation of the case: A healthcare professional (often a doctor or surgeon) presents a detailed summary of the case, including the history, the treatment administered, the patient's progress and any complications that have arisen.

Discussion: The team discusses aspects of the case, asks questions, and identifies areas for improvement or mistakes that may have been made.

Recommendations and action plan: Following the discussion, recommendations are made and an action plan is drawn up to prevent similar events from occurring in the future.

3. A caring and constructive environment

The atmosphere at RMMs must be constructive. The aim is not to blame, but to understand and learn. Goodwill and non-punitivity are essential to encourage the active and honest participation of all members.

4. The importance of documentation

It is crucial to document the discussions and recommendations of MMRs in order to monitor the implementation of improvement actions, but also to keep a record of the discussions for legal or ethical reasons.

5. Disseminating information

The lessons learned from MMRs should not be limited to those who attend them. The lessons must be shared throughout the institution, and even beyond, to ensure continuous improvement in the quality of care.

Morbidity and mortality reviews are an invaluable tool for healthcare establishments wishing to adopt a proactive approach to improving the quality of care. They promote a transparent medical culture focused on collective learning and continuous improvement in patient care.

Chapter 25:
THE EVOLUTION AND CAREER OPPORTUNITIES

Specialisation in internal medicine.

Internal medicine is often described as "adult medicine in all its complexity". It deals with complex or rare diseases that require specific expertise. But what does it really mean to specialise in internal medicine, and why is it so important?

1. Understanding internal medicine
Internal medicine is a medical speciality that focuses on the holistic care of adults. It is not limited to one part of the body or one type of disease, but focuses instead on the diagnosis, treatment and prevention of disease in adults, particularly when several conditions coexist.

2. A rigorous training process
Specialising in internal medicine requires rigorous postgraduate training. After obtaining their medical degree, future internists generally undergo several years of training combining theory, clinical practice, research and sometimes even sub-specialisation in fields such as rheumatology, endocrinology or nephrology.

3. The art of diagnosis
Internists are often seen as "medical detectives". Thanks to their extensive training, they are able to solve complex or enigmatic medical cases. Specialising in internal medicine therefore provides the tools needed to make accurate diagnoses, even in the most confusing situations.

4. Managing multi-disease conditions
With increasing life expectancy, many patients present with several chronic conditions at the same time. Thanks to

their holistic training, internists are particularly well placed to manage these multi-disease cases.

5. Multidisciplinary collaboration
The complex nature of internal medicine means that internists often work closely with other specialists. This can include surgeons, radiologists, pharmacists and even mental health specialists.

6. Research and innovation
Internal medicine is at the forefront of medical research. Many internists are actively involved in clinical research, helping to advance medical knowledge and improve care for all.

7. Sub-specialisations
Over the years, some internists may choose to focus even more on a particular area of internal medicine, becoming experts in fields such as immunology, cardiology or infectious diseases.

Specialising in Internal Medicine is a deep commitment to understanding and treating medical complexity. It is a demanding but rewarding path, with the potential to change the lives of patients facing complex medical challenges.

Research and innovation.

Since its origins, medicine has been a constantly evolving field. It is thanks to research and innovation that major advances have been made, extending the length and quality of life of millions of people. In the context of internal medicine, research and innovation play a vital role, shaping the medical landscape and offering new perspectives on care.

1. A relentless quest for knowledge
Medical research is the foundation on which all advances in medicine are built. It provides answers to fundamental questions, gives us a better understanding of disease mechanisms, and guides the development of new therapies. In internal medicine, with its broad spectrum of diseases, research is omnipresent, from epidemiological studies to clinical trials.

2. The era of personalised medicine
Technological innovation, particularly in genomics, has paved the way for personalised medicine. Thanks to advances in research, it is now possible to tailor treatments to each patient's genetic profile. This tailor-made approach improves the effectiveness of treatments while reducing side effects.

3. Technologies for diagnosis
Innovation is not just pharmacological. Ever more precise and rapid diagnostic equipment is regularly being developed, providing internists with essential tools for making accurate diagnoses. Medical imaging, for example, has undergone major revolutions with techniques such as functional MRI and positron emission tomography (PET).

4. Digitalising healthcare
The digital age has brought its share of innovations, including electronic medical records, telemedicine and medical applications. These tools facilitate communication, patient monitoring and access to information, making care more efficient and appropriate.

5. Interdisciplinary collaboration
The complex challenges of modern medicine require a collaborative approach. Innovation often comes from the fusion of skills from different fields: biologists, chemists, computer scientists, engineers and doctors join forces to design tomorrow's solutions.

6. The ethical challenges of innovation
Every medical advance raises its own set of ethical questions. Research and innovation must therefore always

be conducted with caution, taking into account the moral and societal implications of discoveries.

Research and innovation in internal medicine are more vital than ever. They are the driving force behind the development of care, enabling us to meet the medical challenges of today and tomorrow. Every discovery, every innovation, strengthens the therapeutic arsenal of internists and opens up new prospects for patients around the world.

Ongoing training.

In medicine, the only constant is change. As technologies evolve, new research sheds new light and diseases change, healthcare professionals are called upon to adapt. At the heart of this evolution is continuing education, ensuring that practitioners remain at the cutting edge of their field and offer the highest quality care.

1. Responding to a changing medical world
Medicine is not static. Between technological developments, scientific discoveries and new clinical recommendations, information from ten years ago can become obsolete or even erroneous. Continuing education enables professionals to remain informed and competent in their day-to-day practice.

2. Strengthening clinical excellence
Regular updating of clinical skills is essential to ensure quality care. For example, new surgical techniques or innovative therapeutic approaches can significantly improve patient outcomes. Familiarising yourself with these advances through continuing education is essential for any professional committed to excellence.

3. Cultivating multidisciplinarity
Internal medicine is, by its very nature, an interdisciplinary field. Continuing education offers internists the opportunity

to learn about related specialities, fostering a better overall understanding of the patient and a holistic approach to care.

4. Adapting to regulatory and ethical developments

Beyond the purely clinical aspects, medicine is governed by constantly evolving regulatory and ethical standards. Continuing training enables healthcare professionals to keep abreast of the latest guidelines, thereby ensuring that their practice is both compliant and ethical.

5. Promoting research and innovation

Taking part in training courses can also stimulate interest in clinical research, encouraging professionals to get involved in studies, test new approaches or collaborate with experts in other fields.

6. Professional well-being

In addition to technical skills, continuing training can also cover aspects such as stress management, patient-caregiver communication and work-life balance. This training is crucial to guaranteeing the well-being of carers and, ultimately, the quality of the care delivered.

Continuing education is much more than just a professional obligation. It is a commitment to excellence, a promise to patients and a recognition of the intrinsic dynamism of medicine. In internal medicine, a vast and complex field, this commitment takes on particular importance, guaranteeing modern, ethical and high-quality care.

Conclusion:

The future of internal medicine and the role of the nurse.

By its very nature, internal medicine encompasses a wide variety of pathologies and clinical situations. At the crossroads of several specialities, it is at the forefront of medical, technological and societal developments. While the internist is often seen as the conductor of this vast discipline, the nurse plays the invaluable role of central pillar, guaranteeing the fluidity and efficiency of care. On the eve of new medical revolutions, how is internal medicine set to evolve, and what role will nurses play?

1. Faced with an ageing population
With increasing life expectancy, more and more elderly patients are coming into internal medicine, often suffering from several diseases at the same time. In this context, nurses play a crucial role in the overall care of these patients, combining technical skills with listening and humanity.

2. The rise of new technologies
Telemedicine, artificial intelligence and connected devices are revolutionising the way in which healthcare is delivered. Nurses are in the front line when it comes to integrating these tools into their practice, ensuring high-quality transmission of information and guaranteeing optimum use for the benefit of the patient.

3. A patient-centred approach
Increasingly, medicine is becoming personalised, taking into account not only the disease but also, and above all, the patient as a whole. The nurse, through his or her privileged and constant contact with the patient, becomes the guarantor of this holistic approach, taking care to consider the individual before the pathology.

4. Changing skills and responsibilities
The modern nurse is a far cry from the stereotypical image of the past. Equipped with advanced skills, they are called upon to work closely with the internist, taking an active part in establishing the diagnosis, implementing the care plan and evaluating the results. This increased responsibility requires appropriate, in-depth continuing training.

5. Facing societal challenges
From ethical issues to the challenges posed by health inequalities, not to mention the need for transparent and respectful communication, nurses are often on the front line. Their role extends far beyond technical care, making them a major player in the relationship between patient and carer and a pillar of trust between hospital and patient.

The future of internal medicine is taking shape every day, driven by constant advances and the challenges of a changing society. At the heart of these developments, nurses are steadily strengthening their role, affirming their essential place within the medical team. More than just an operator, nurses are the guarantors of humane, effective and forward-looking medicine.

The importance of adaptation and continuous updating.

In a world as dynamic and evolving as that of healthcare, adapting and updating skills is not only recommended, it is vital. While the primary vocation of medicine is to treat, to remain relevant it must also embrace the technological, scientific and societal changes that are constantly shaping it.

1. A constantly changing medical world

Medicine is a field in which innovations are emerging at a frenetic pace. New diseases are emerging, old protocols are being called into question, revolutionary treatments are being discovered, and cutting-edge technologies are being developed. In the face of this relentless dynamic, to remain static is to fall behind, or even become obsolete.

2. Improved quality of care

Continuous adaptation and updating enables healthcare professionals to offer better quality care. By keeping abreast of the latest advances, they can adopt best practice, minimising the risks to patients while maximising the chances of therapeutic success.

3. The importance of medical ethics

Developments in knowledge and technology raise new ethical dilemmas. It is therefore crucial for healthcare professionals to keep abreast of ethical debates and discussions so that they can make informed decisions that respect patients' dignity and rights.

4. Patient confidence

Patients are increasingly well informed and have access to a plethora of information via the internet. They rightly expect their carer to be at the cutting edge of knowledge. Continuous adaptation and updating are therefore essential to maintain patient confidence and strengthen the therapeutic relationship.

5. A professional and personal challenge

Beyond the purely medical aspect, continuous adaptation is also a professional and personal development issue. It enables carers to remain motivated, committed and passionate about their work. It also gives them the opportunity to develop their careers, take on new responsibilities and achieve their full potential.

Continuous adaptation and updating are not just fashionable concepts in the medical world. They reflect a deep commitment to the vocation of care. By embracing these principles, healthcare professionals not only ensure the best possible care for their patients, they also guarantee themselves a rich, progressive and deeply satisfying career.

Glossary of medical terms.

Case history: Collection and analysis of information provided by the patient about his/her medical history and that of his/her family.

Antibiotic: Drug used to treat bacterial infections.

Benign: Not life-threatening. This is often opposed to "malignant", a terminology frequently used for tumours or cancers.

Catheter: thin, flexible tube inserted into a blood vessel or body cavity to administer or withdraw fluids.

Decompensation: worsening of a chronic illness.

Etiology: Study of the causes of a disease.

Haemorrhage: Abnormally heavy loss of blood.

Inflammation: Reaction of the body to an injury or infection, generally characterised by redness, heat, swelling and pain.

Lesion: Alteration of tissue caused by disease or trauma.

Metastasis: Spread of a disease, particularly cancer, from its site of origin to other parts of the body.

Neuropathy: Disease or dysfunction of the nerves.

Oncology: Branch of medicine that studies and treats cancer.

Pathology: Study of diseases.

Remission: Reduction or disappearance of the signs and symptoms of an illness.

Symptom: Manifestation of a disease or disorder experienced by a patient.

Tachycardia: Acceleration of the heart rate.

Ulcer: open, often painful lesion that forms on the skin or mucous membranes.

Vaccine: Substance introduced into the body to induce immunity against a specific disease.

Xeno-: Prefix meaning "foreign", as in xenograft (transplantation of organs from one species to another).

Zoonosis: Disease transmissible from animals to humans.

This glossary is far from complete, as the medical field is vast and constantly evolving. It is always useful to consult a specialised medical dictionary or a health professional for precise, up-to-date definitions.

Additional resources for continuing education.

Continuing education is essential for healthcare professionals to keep up to date with the latest advances, methods and medical protocols. Here is a list of resources to help professionals continue their training:

- Professional associations and trade unions :
    - National Order of Nurses.
    - Society of Internal Medicine.
    - Collège National des Généralistes Enseignants.
- Conferences and workshops :
    - National and international conferences related to internal medicine or the specialty concerned.
    - Practical workshops to improve certain skills.
- Newspapers and medical journals :
    - The Lancet
    - New England Journal of Medicine
    - Journal of Internal Medicine
- Universities and medical schools :
    - Continuing education modules offered by academic institutions.
    - Master's and PhD programmes for further specialisation.
- Online courses :
    - Sites such as Coursera, Udemy and EdX offer specialist courses in many medical fields.
    - MOOCs (Massive Open Online Courses) offered by leading academic institutions.
- Books and e-books :
    - Recent publications on specific subjects.
    - Manuals of general and specialist medicine.
- Medical applications :

Applications such as UpToDate, Medscape and Epocrates offer up-to-date information on diseases, medicines and more.

Webinars :

Online seminars offered by experts on topical or specialist subjects.

Professional social networks :

Networks such as ResearchGate or LinkedIn allow you to follow the latest news and research from the medical community.

Simulations and virtual reality:

Innovative tools for practising procedures in a virtual environment.

Competence and training centres :

Institutions that offer practical training, workshops and simulations to hone skills.

Certification bodies :

Organisations that offer certification in specialist areas, attesting to mastery of a subject or skill.

It is essential that healthcare professionals take responsibility for their own continuing education. This not only improves their skills and knowledge, but also boosts the confidence of their patients and the quality of the care they provide.

www.ingramcontent.com/pod-product-compliance
Lightning Source LLC
Chambersburg PA
CBHW072157290526
45794CB00004B/1553